KU-675-007

GOOD HEALTH

breasts

your 100 questions answered

Liz Bestic
Claire Gillman

Newleaf

First published by

NEWLEAF

an imprint of

GILL & MACMILLAN LTD

Hume Avenue, Park West, Dublin 12

with associated companies throughout the world

www.gillmacmillan.ie

ISBN 0 7171 3271 4

A CIP catalogue record for this book is available from the British Library.

Note from the publisher
Information given in this book is not intended to be
taken as a replacement for medical advice. Any person with
a condition requiring medical attention should consult a
qualified medical practitioner or therapist.

This book was conceived, designed and produced by
THE IVY PRESS LIMITED

ART DIRECTOR Peter Bridgewater
PUBLISHER Sophie Collins
EDITORIAL DIRECTOR Steve Luck
DESIGNER Jane Lanaway
PROJECT EDITOR Georga Godwin
DTP DESIGNER Chris Lanaway
MEDICAL ILLUSTRATOR Michael Courtney

Printed in Spain by Graficomo, S.A.

Contents

Introduction

Love them or hate them, breasts are here to stay. Whether yours come in a small but perfectly formed 32AA cup or a more voluptuous 38DD, you have probably by now formed a lasting relationship with them. Never before have we lived in an age when breasts are so in-your-face, so to speak.

From the first day a woman sprouts breasts, her life is never the same again. Not only is she bombarded with a whole range of media images of what society thinks her breasts should look like, but an army of experts starts telling her what to do with them. So should she wear a bra, or will it cause her cancer? Should she feed her baby herself, or resort to formula milk? She will fret at every new health scare and agonize endlessly over whether her breasts are too large or too small, and whether her lover/partner/husband really likes them.

As a pubescent girl at school, she may be ribbed mercilessly by teenage boys. Most youths at this age are breast-obsessed and consider it a great wheeze to poke fun at a girl's breasts, calling them a litany of unsavoury names, from tits,

A view that isn't normally seen: a cross section of a healthy breast showing milk ducts and component tissue.

Muscle

Fat

Reservoirs

Mammary gland (alveoli)

jugs and jars to boobs, bouncers and bazookas. If she survives secondary school with her dignity intact and her self-confidence still in place, she faces college and the world of work, with its attendant sexist comments and outmoded dress codes.

Women are constantly bombarded with conflicting messages. On the one hand, we're encouraged to be able to slip effortlessly into a size-10 shift dress; on the other, countless advertising images tell us that 36D full bosoms are the order of the day. In fact, so closely is a big bust linked to desirability that it took less than 12 months for *Baywatch* babe Pamela Anderson to lose her top spot on the Internet charts after she had her breast implants removed. Unfeasibly large though her enhanced bust may have been, it seems that this was the main reason for her popularity with the Net-surfing members of the opposite sex.

Yet if you ask women themselves about the perfect bust, surveys reveal that most of us believe that a modest 34C is ideal and anything larger seems increasingly unattractive.

In a survey to identify the best breasts in show business, Geri Halliwell came top. The former Spice Girl beat off stiff competition from Jennifer Lopez, Elle MacPherson and Liz Hurley to win the honour.

As we can see, most women rate their breasts by comparing them with other people's – complete folly though this may be, because there is no 'perfect' breast – so it may take many years to accept them the way they are. Indeed, for many women it is not until they have their first child and discover that their breasts actually fulfil a useful purpose that they shed their inhibitions. Suddenly the penny drops and they are amazed that their breasts more than adequately nurture and feed their babies.

Unfortunately, no sooner do we feel comfortable with our bosoms than age and post-pregnancy shrinkage start to take effect and we again become dissatisfied with our droopy breasts. That is probably why about 40,000 American women get breast implants each year, at an average surgeon's fee (add hospital and anaesthesia bills) of $2700* (£1860). Mind you, a further 36,000 are paying $4700* (£3240) for a breast reduction each year, so it seems that – whatever nature endows us with – we are not satisfied. (*Figures from the American Society of Plastic and Reconstructive Surgeons.)

Breasts through history
Breasts have not always been such a source of dismay to women. Throughout history women were usually depicted in art with their breasts exposed. Even in the Christian Church females were painted with one or more breasts uncovered: if proof were needed, just take a look at the Sistine Chapel. In

fact, down the ages breasts have been represented as symbols of woman, who is both full-breasted nurturer and pre-pubescent virgin at one and the same time.

In the seventeenth and eighteenth centuries breasts were also seen as a symbol of power. Many artists depicted bare-breasted women boldly leading their troops into battle. Marianne, the symbol of France, was one of these brave warriors and is often seen in paintings striding through the battlefield inciting the revolutionaries to fight on. She was viewed as a 'total woman', but her breasts represented more than a mere symbol of power – according to tradition they literally fed the troops with the milk they contained!

It is also worth noting that right up until the nineteenth century women with sufficient means paid for their babies to be breastfed by a nursing mother of lower status than themselves. This woman was known as a wet-nurse, and the practice was widespread in Europe from medieval times. There is even some evidence that in classical Greece and Rome female domestic slaves acted as wet-nurses. They often lived with the family, rather than the family farming the baby out to a wet-nurse, as became the custom later on in Europe.

In many cultures there was – and still is – a taboo on having sex while lactating. The growth in the popularity of wet-nursing was probably as much to do with husbands demanding the sexual services of their wives as soon as possible after childbirth as it was to do with women opting out of their maternal duties. Wet-nursing finally died out in Britain at the end of the eighteenth century, although in France it carried on right up to the advent of bottle-feeding at the end of the nineteenth century.

It was not until the repressive Victorian era that female breasts and sexuality finally became strongly connected. During this period women were expected to cover more of their bodies, although, para-doxically, their clothing was carefully designed to accentuate and expose their breasts, stopping just short of actually showing any nipple.

From that time on, in Western society, the female breast's status as an object of attraction and as a sexual icon was assured.

Breasts through fashion

It was not until the invention of the bra that breasts really came into their own as a fashion statement. The brassière literally burst onto the scene in the 1920s, releasing women from the confines of the corset, which had encased their bust, waist and hips.

Nobody is quite sure who 'invented' the bra and many people have laid claim to the idea. One story has it that in 1913 Mary Phelps Jacobs, a wealthy New York débutante, was being dressed by her French maid for a ball. Her corset was firmly outlined through her diaphanous gown, so Mary was set to wear nothing at all underneath. Suddenly she and her maid hit upon the idea of combining two handkerchiefs and some ribbon into what resembles today's halterneck top. Mary patented her idea in 1914 and called it a 'backless brassière'. She popularized her design by sending samples to all her socialite friends and finally sold it to the Warner Brothers Corset Company for $1500 (£1035).

In 1922 a forward-thinking woman named Ida Rosenthal picked up and ran with the idea. She was a visionary who saw beyond the flat-chested, boyish look that was so popular with the 'flappers' of the 1920s and early 1930s. She predicted a time when curves would be 'in' again and led the move towards sized bras. The industry standard of A–D cups, which we continue to use today, was started by the Warner Company in 1935.

The 1920s and 1930s saw a greater sexual focus on legs and backs. During the Second World War, however, Rosenthal's predictions proved correct, as pin-ups sent to the soldiers at the front featured women who were anything but boyish, the most notable being Betty Grable. After the war the breast reigned supreme until the 1960s, reaching heights of admiration never previously attained.

By the 1950s the Hollywood sex queen was an established icon, and women all over the developed world were heavily influenced by Hollywood dress code and attitudes. The 'bullet bra' hit the scene at about the same time as the buxom Hollywood sex starlets reached their pinnacle. Women such as

Marilyn Monroe and Jane Mansfield made the equation that 'large breasts equals sexy' easy for everyone to understand.

The late 1950s also saw the first publication of top-shelf titles such as *Playboy* magazine. Until this time the only pictures of uncovered breasts that could be seen were either in technical journals (usually line drawings) or in *National Geographic* (depicting native tribes). With the advent of men's magazines and Hollywood starlets, young males were exposed to female breasts as never before and a new definition of sex appeal was established. As most of the actresses and models in vogue were large-breasted a big bust became synonymous with sex appeal, a notion that has never quite gone away.

Simultaneously bras began to lose their role as functional items of dress and become fashion accessories. That is, until the 1960s, when the feminists famously burned theirs. For a short time the bra was considered an item of male oppression and, contrary to intention, the bra-less period of liberation was undoubtedly welcomed by male breast-admirers everywhere. However, no sooner were the flames dying down than the 'Cross-your-heart bra' was invented, closely followed by the 'Wonderbra', both a godsend to women who were less than well-endowed.

In the 1980s Madonna took us back to the Dark Ages with her conical bra designed by Jean-Paul Gaultier, but for women who felt bras were built for comfort the emergence of the sports bra was a salvation. And in 1994 bras stood accused of murder: *Dressed to Kill* was a controversial book, which suggested that wearing bras inhibited the function of the lymphatic system in and around the breasts; the resulting build-up of toxins supposingly causing cancer. The theory has since been disproved. Women now have a bemusing array of uplift, maximizer and minimizer bras from which to choose, while the millennium promises us new technology that is developing plastic breasts to insert into our bras.

Cultural differences

Preoccupation with the bra as a fashion statement – and, indeed, with the sexuality of breasts themselves – is far from universal. There are widespread cultural differences throughout the world in men's and women's attitudes towards breasts and the role they play in sexual attraction. In some societies breasts are rarely covered, while Eastern and Western attitudes to the female form vary considerably. In Arab culture an ample bosom is not nearly as important as voluptuous thighs and buttocks. For Hindus, the body is cherished and each part has an important role to play in sexual relations. In Islam a woman must cloak herself from head to toe to cover all her body because female sexuality is perceived as dangerous. Meanwhile, on the beaches of the Mediterranean, women routinely go topless.

How to use this book

Despite the high profile role that breasts enjoy in modern society, mystery still surrounds them and sorting fact from folklore is not easy. For example, despite what advertisers would have us believe, big breasts don't necessarily mean more fun. As breasts are most sensitive around the nipples there is no reason why women with large breasts should get more sexual satisfaction than the less well-endowed.

This book draws together the 100 questions that women most commonly ask about the health, function and care of their breasts. The book is split into four sections, covering breasts in general, breasts during pregnancy and breastfeeding, breast cancer and, finally, cosmetic breast surgery.

You may simply want to know about general maintenance and what sort of bra to choose, or you may want to understand what happens during treatment for breast cancer. Decisions about whether to breast- or bottle-feed, and whether to enhance your body by surgery, will all be made easier if you are better informed. The information in this book will help you to make your own informed decisions.

Whether you are ambivalent about your bust or love your breasts to bits, it is important to know what you can do to keep them in tiptop shape and functioning properly. This guide will help you to live comfortably with your breasts (whatever size or shape nature gave you) and – if there are problems – information on where to seek help.

Prevention

*Throughout your life your breasts undergo
a range of changes. A basic knowledge
of what makes them function and how they are
affected by puberty, pregnancy, breastfeeding
and the menopause will help you understand
these changes and how to deal with any
problems that may arise.*

My mother tells me that I should spend as much as I can afford on a bra and to make sure that it fits well. I have heard that bras can cause breast cancer and think it may be better not to wear one at all. If I do wear a bra, how important is it to have a well-fitting one, and will I have saggy breasts when I'm older if I don't wear one?

There is no evidence to suggest that there is any link between wearing a bra and breast cancer. There is, however, evidence to suggest that wearing a bra may exacerbate breast pain in women who are prone to it. Some research has even shown that wearing a bra makes no difference at all to the firmness of your breasts, because gravity will win out in the end!

Whatever you believe, most women do end up wearing a bra, particularly if they have large breasts. Breasts contain fat and glands but no muscle, so many experts think it is important to prevent the ligaments that provide natural support from overstretching. Good support, especially during exercise or when playing sports, stops the breasts from jiggling up and down.

When choosing a bra, the important thing is to make sure that it has adjustable straps and fittings, and that it gives the correct amount of support. When you try on a bra, do some normal movements like bending and stretching to make sure that it does not ride up or become uncomfortable.

Cup sizes generally range from AA (which is small) to DD (large), but some specialists make bras up to a GG fitting. Many women have one breast larger than the other, so always fit the larger one when choosing a bra. Check that the bra lies flat around your body and is not too tight or causes any breathing difficulties. Your breasts should be fully contained within each cup. Gaping at the side means that the cup is too small, while if the cup wrinkles all over it means that it is too large. If the bra has underwiring, then the side should lie flat against your body, following its contours, rather than digging into your breast. If you have a heavy bust, the bra straps should be wide and strong enough to support it. Always test the fit of a bra while both standing and sitting, as the breast tends to 'plump up' when you are seated.

A well-fitting bra with the correct cup size provides good support. If you are in any doubt about your size, ask to be measured in your local department store. Many lingerie departments have experienced staff who can measure you and fit you with a comfortable bra in exactly the right size.

A well-fitting bra is essential for your comfort and support. Most lingerie departments offer a fitting service and it is a good idea to have your size checked regularly.

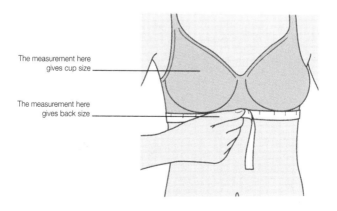

The measurement here gives cup size

The measurement here gives back size

I went to buy a bra last week and was bemused by the array of choice. I guess that I'm an average bust size. Is there any particular merit in the various styles?

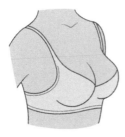

The push up bra gives you a movie-star cleavage.

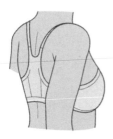

The sports bra gives extra support, and not just whilst exercising.

Yes, the different styles do have particular merits. Research shows that 75 per cent of women are wearing the wrong-sized bra because they have never in their lives undergone a proper fitting. Experts believe that it is important to be fitted every single time you buy a bra, unless you are buying an exact repeat of the style that you had before. There are bras for running, for sports, for going out, for wearing to the office, for the evening and for the bedroom. You may even need a different bra for the time of the month when your breasts feel heavier. You can have different bras for different occasions, just as you have different shoes. However, most people just buy a bra off the shelf, thinking that if they were 34B 20 years ago, then they must still be the same size now.

Sports bras are good if you do a lot of exercise. If you are thinking of buying a sports bra, it may amuse you to know that the very first one was invented by two American women in 1977 – by sewing together two jockstraps! Fortunately things have progressed since then, and there is now a host of shapes and styles to choose from. Experts say that the ideal sports bra is one that feels like a second skin. The most important features to look out for are good support, strong sides, a wide back and adjustable straps. And some modern fabrics literally

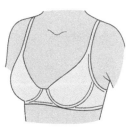

The underwired bra is the most popular. It combines good support with a fashionable look.

draw moisture away from the skin, rather like a baby's nappy. There are two basic types of sports bra: compression ones (suitable for women with small-to-medium busts), which work by pushing the breasts down; and more conventional-style bras, which support the bust.

In general terms if you have large, heavy breasts, then you require a bra with wide straps, good support and probably underwiring. The smaller bust can cope with seamless bras that offer less support. The bust can be made to look bigger with specially designed uplift or balcony bras. ●

I have very small breasts and worry that when I have a baby I may not be able to feed it. Is there any correlation between large breasts and milk production?

There is no correlation at all between breast size and milk production. Larger breasts have a higher proportion of fatty tissue, compared to glandular tissue, but this has no effect on the amount of milk you produce. You do not need to worry that because of small breasts you will be unable to nourish your baby. It is rare for a woman to be born with insufficient glandular tissue. Interestingly, women with small breasts often have fewer difficulties than bigger-busted women as positioning when breastfeeding often presents challenges for mothers with large breasts (*see Q 25*). ●

Q

4 My daughter is only 12, but she has started growing breasts already. How important is it for her to wear a bra this early on in her development, and where should I go to get her fitted?

When teenagers first start to develop breasts it can be a very exciting time for them. They often want to wear a bra long before they are really ready. There is absolutely no harm in your daughter being fitted for her first bra, but there are one or two things you should remember.

When choosing a bra for your daughter, make sure that it has adjustable straps and fittings and gives the correct amount of support. If the straps cut into her shoulder, she may need wider straps or underwiring. The cups of the bra should lift and separate the breasts. The bra should lie flat around the body and not dig into the flesh. Any bulging at the armpits means that the side panels may be too narrow. If in doubt, ask for expert advice from a fitting specialist.

Your daughter may not always need to buy the same bra size – styles and makes vary considerably. If her breasts are a different size or get bigger just before her period, then stretch bras may be more comfortable. Many teenagers like to wear underwired bras because they make them feel more grown-up. Be particularly careful to choose an underwired bra that fits correctly – a badly fitting bra can cause pain and discomfort if the wires dig into the upper part of the breast. The more expensive underwired bras tend to contain softer, more flexible wires.

5 My nipples go very hard and erect when I am sexually aroused. Why is this?

The nipples are a particularly sensitive erogenous zone for women. They contain sensory nerves that carry signals such as touch, pain and temperature. Each breast has an abundant supply of these nerves, which are responsible for the sensitivity of the areola (the skin around the nipple) and the nipple itself. Breasts also contain nerves from the autonomic nervous system, which controls involuntary body functions, and this is what causes the connection between nipple stimulation and arousal in the genital area and orgasm.

During sexual arousal the breasts become up to 25 per cent bigger. Tiny muscle fibres in the nipple contract, increasing both the length and diameter of the nipple. When the nipples become erect, the surrounding areolae grow darker. You may even notice a pink flush extending over the front of your body, especially across the breasts. This is caused by dilated blood vessels and increased blood flow, and is known as a sexual flush.

As you get older, swelling of the breasts during sexual excitement gradually diminishes because of the loss of breast tissue. By the age of 50, although nipple erection still occurs, only about one-fifth of women experience an increase in breast size similar to that when they were younger.

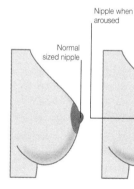

Nipple when aroused

Normal sized nipple

Your breasts become up to 25 per cent bigger when you are sexually aroused. This is most noticeable in your nipples, which, for many, are a major source of sexual pleasure.

I suffer from painful, swollen breasts before and during my periods. Is this normal?

This is very normal indeed. Around five million women in the UK are known to suffer from breast pain – or mastalgia, as it is sometimes called. And a recent survey showed that 70 per cent of women had experienced breast pain at some time in their life. Where breast pain is not severe, many women manage to accept it as a normal and temporary feature of the changes that occur during their menstrual cycle. Breast pain rarely signals anything more sinister, particularly as breast cancer itself is normally painless.

There are two types of breast pain: cyclical and non-cyclical. If you don't know whether your breast pain follows any particular pattern, then it may be worth keeping a diary for a couple of months. Cyclical breast pain is the sort of pain that occurs once a month, usually three to seven days before your period. Many women notice that their breasts seem heavy or uncomfortably tender at this time of the month and just learn to live with it. As you grow older, particularly when you reach your thirties, you may find that this tenderness becomes more like real pain. This often also happens when older women go on to hormone replacement therapy (HRT), but usually disappears with the end of the menopause.

You may find that the pain is not the same every month or that certain movements increase your

BREAST PAIN

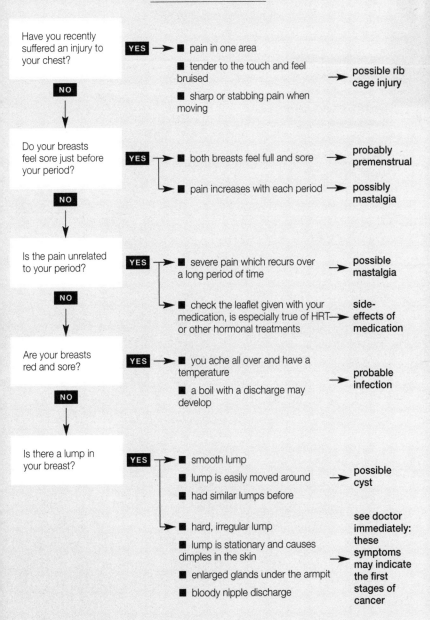

Have you recently suffered an injury to your chest?

YES →
- pain in one area
- tender to the touch and feel bruised → **possible rib cage injury**
- sharp or stabbing pain when moving

NO ↓

Do your breasts feel sore just before your period?

YES →
- both breasts feel full and sore → **probably premenstrual**
- pain increases with each period → **possibly mastalgia**

NO ↓

Is the pain unrelated to your period?

YES →
- severe pain which recurs over a long period of time → **possible mastalgia**
- check the leaflet given with your medication, is especially true of HRT or other hormonal treatments → **side-effects of medication**

NO ↓

Are your breasts red and sore?

YES →
- you ache all over and have a temperature → **probable infection**
- a boil with a discharge may develop

NO ↓

Is there a lump in your breast?

YES →
- smooth lump
- lump is easily moved around → **possible cyst**
- had similar lumps before

- hard, irregular lump
- lump is stationary and causes dimples in the skin
- enlarged glands under the armpit → **see doctor immediately: these symptoms may indicate the first stages of cancer**
- bloody nipple discharge

discomfort. Nobody really knows what causes non-cyclical breast pain, although some women have been found to have abnormal levels of certain fatty acids in their blood; or it may be that particular lifestyle factors, such as smoking, intake of caffeine and diet, play a role.

For around 15 per cent of women, breast pain is severe enough to disrupt their lives. If you are in this category your doctor may suggest a course of evening-primrose oil. Some women respond very well to this and their breast pain never returns. If your pain does not respond, then there are drug treatments that block the release of hormones from the pituitary gland (at the base of the skull), reduce the amount of hormones produced by the ovaries and the quantity of circulating oestrogen, which exacerbates breast pain. Other drugs interfere with oestrogen by stopping it reaching its target cells.

If you are taking the contraceptive pill, your doctor may suggest changing from one brand to another or stopping the pill for a few months to see if there are any changes in your symptoms. Ironically, if you are not on the pill, your doctor may well suggest it as a solution to the problem! Some health experts recommend a change of diet, cutting down on caffeine and reducing your intake of meat and dairy products if you suffer from breast pain. ●

Budding

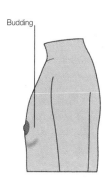

My teenage daughter has been the butt of inappropriate sexual innuendo from boys because of her large chest and prominent nipples. This makes her very self-conscious. What advice should I give her?

Very large breasts can cause young women a lot of problems. You need to reassure your daughter that breasts come in all sorts of shapes and sizes and that she may well like her large breasts as she gets older. If they are causing a real problem because of the embarrassment factor, talk the subject over with your doctor. Sometimes large breasts are painful or their weight causes backache. If your daughter is really worried by them, and she has reached an age when she has stopped growing, it may be possible for her to have an operation called a reduction mammoplasty (see Q 53) to reduce their size. The operation is no longer considered purely cosmetic, doctors are more aware of the effect that large breasts can have on physical and psychological well-being. The benefits from the operation are often dramatic and worthwhile, but she should be aware that such an operation may affect her ability to breastfeed later on.

Starting to grow

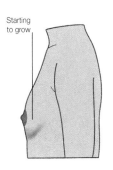

Fully formed

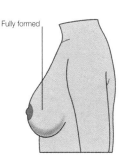

There is no knowing how fast, how big or quite when a woman's breasts will grow. Some girls can become full and curvy whilst their friends seem never to catch up.

8 I've read conflicting advice in the press regarding whether or not stress can trigger breast cancer. Have scientists come to a consensus yet?

Researchers say that the link between stress and relapse among breast-cancer patients remains unsolved. However, a recent British study disputes the theory that stress can trigger breast cancer by accelerating the growth of cancer cells. The study of 332 women showed that those who had been diagnosed with breast cancer were no more likely to have experienced stress than those with a benign lump. The researchers argue that stressful life events are common to everyone, with approximately two-thirds of women with breast lumps (both benign and malignant) experiencing at least one highly stressful life event in the previous five years. However, this study contradicts the results of earlier research, which concluded that extreme stress *can* trigger breast cancer – those researchers found that women who reported severe stress in the previous five years were 50 per cent more likely to have breast cancer than those experiencing less acute stress.

I've read about the breast-screening programme that is available for women. Why is breast-screening so important?

Women are much better informed and educated on health issues today than our parents' generation was. From 1940 to 1982 there was a steady rise in the incidence of breast cancer and this was attributed to a gradual increase in the underlying risk factors, such as delayed childbearing and having fewer children. However, there is now a greater detection rate for breast cancer, due to breast-screening programmes and the greater use of self-examination. Mortality rates are dropping as a combined result of better and earlier detection of the disease and an improvement in cancer treatments.

In the UK, where breast cancer kills 1,000 every month, 1.4 million women have an annual mammogram on the national screening programme. The programme has contributed to a 21 per cent drop in deaths from the disease in England and Wales over the last ten years. In Ireland there is a new screening programme where women aged 50 and over are called in for a mammograph. Researchers believe that the death rate should fall even more over the next decade, as more women are screened. Early detection is the key to improving the chances of recovery from breast cancer: when detected in its earliest stage, the disease is 90 per cent curable. And remember: breast-screening starts with self-examination (*see Q 13*).

10 My mother is full-bosomed, but I have very small breasts. What determines the size of a woman's bust?

The size of your breasts, like your overall appearance, is genetically determined. Normally, if your mother has a large bust, then you may well follow suit. However, small breasts must also be in your family's genes – perhaps on your father's side, or further back in your mother's family.

Once developed, your breasts can fluctuate in size in response to changes in your weight, pregnancy and breastfeeding. They can also vary slightly throught your menstruation cycle. As you get older the shape of your breasts also changes. Unfortunately this is usually in the form of a gradual drooping. Most women have breasts of slightly different size and, in some cases, there is a very clear difference between them. ●

Breasts come in all shapes and sizes. Whilst this is determined by genes it does not follow that you will take after your mother.

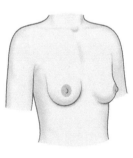

Small breasts are just as capable as large breasts at fulfilling their biological functions.

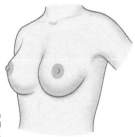

Large breasted women often complain about the discomfort and unwanted attention they attract.

I have heard that you shouldn't scrub the breasts or use any beauty treatments on them. How are you supposed to make sure the skin stays soft and supple and the nipples in good condition?

The skin of the breasts is very delicate and should be treated carefully. Try not to scrub or dry your breasts roughly with a towel, since this can make the nipples sore and tender. If your nipples do become dry and flaky (as often happens just before a period), moisturize them twice a week with a fragrance-free moisturizing lotion. If you have inverted nipples, clean them with cotton-wool buds to prevent secretions collecting. Don't squeeze your nipples, as this may increase their secretions and, if you have spots on your breasts, could lead to an infection or an abscess. Always check any moles for signs of changes. If they become bigger, darker or start to bleed, see your doctor right away. You may be advised to have them removed.

Some women develop hair around the nipples, but are quite content with their appearance. However, if this troubles you, remove the hair from around your nipples with tweezers, not a depilatory cream. Permanent hair removal by electrolysis should only be done by a fully trained professional.

If you notice any persistent patches of eczema, go and see your doctor; wear a cotton bra. If you like topless sunbathing, you may be increasing your risk of getting skin cancer. It is important to protect your breasts from the sun's rays: apply a sunblock with a protection factor higher than 15 every two hours.

12 I have been told that there are breast-firming lotions and that I can exercise to tone up my bust. However, my son, who is a gym instructor, tells me that too much exercise can actually cause your breasts to sag. What should I believe, and what can I do to help myself?

There is a grain of truth in both statements. In the old days people believed that the best way to keep your breast pert was to bathe it first in hot water and then in cold water. This did wonders for the areola (the area around the nipple) and made the nipples erect, which may have been mistaken for pertness. The reality, however, is that no amount of potions or lotions will improve the shape or texture of the breasts, since this is determined by your body's response to oestrogens secreted during puberty and then with each menstrual cycle.

Your son is right when he says that exercise can damage your breasts in the long-term. If you work out regularly, you may end up with droopy, wrinkled breasts unless you start taking a few precautions. Breasts can bounce up and down by up to 7cm (2¾in) during exercise, according to recent research, and this can cause irreversible damage.

Help reduce sagging by doing push ups. Kneel on all fours (a) with hands shoulder width apart and palms flat. Stretch each leg out and bend your arms lowering your chest (b). Repeat ten times.

a

b

Breasts are composed entirely of fat and tissue – with no muscle. Constant motion stretches the supporting tissue (known as Cooper's ligaments), which in turn causes sagging. Breasts cannot be toned up in the same way as other parts of your body, because of the lack of muscle, but you can try the following exercises to work on your pectoral muscles, since keeping these firm gives added support to the Cooper's ligaments.

Try pressing your palms together in front of your breasts (c). Hold for five seconds, relax and then repeat the exercise ten times. Alternatively, grasp your forearms at shoulder level and then pull them outwards without letting go (d). Repeat 10–15 times. Finally, curl your fingers and interlock them at shoulder height, then try to pull them apart (e). Hold for five seconds, then repeat the exercise 10–15 times.

The other thing you can do to delay long-term sagging is to ensure that you always wear a proper sports bra as this can halve the amount of breast motion. Even women with small breasts need to be supported, as research shows that if you wear an A cup, your breast movement still ranges up to 4.2cm (1½in) away from the control point on the body, when not supported. In fact, some experts recommend that you wear a sports bra even for low-impact physical work.

Exercises (c), (d) and (e) are designed to strengthen the pectoral muscles which can take some of the strain off the Cooper's ligaments and so help to keep your breasts pert.

c
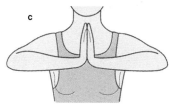

d
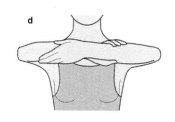

e
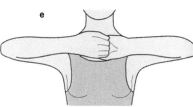

Q

13 I am 17 and have not yet begun to examine my breasts. Am I too young to start, and what exactly should I be looking for?

The first stage of the breast examination is to examine them in a mirror. As you get to know the way they look you can easily recognize when something is not quite right.

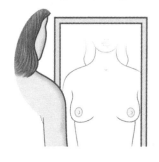

You are never too young to start examining your breasts. As soon as you start your periods is a good time to familiarize yourself with your breasts. Then you can start to recognize any changes that take place during your menstrual cycle.

Start by looking at your breasts in the mirror. Study each one for changes in size, appearance, colour of the nipples and differences in level between the nipples. If there is any sign of eczema or dimpling of the skin you should seek medical advice. You will also be able to tell over time whether it is normal for your breasts to become more lumpy during the second half of your menstrual cycle.

After the visual examination, lie down with one arm behind your head and feel your breasts with your fingertips. Using a firm touch, examine your right breast with your left hand. Check all the way up into your armpit and along the top of your collarbone for lumps that could be swollen

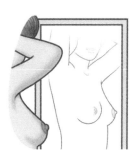
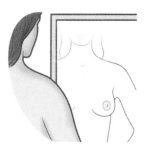
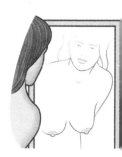

lymph nodes. Do the same with your right hand on your left breast. Once you have examined your breasts a few times you will begin to know what is normal for you.

As you begin to know your own breasts, you can be alert to any changes that might require a visit to your doctor. You can check for nipple discharge by examining your clothes. This is only significant if it appears without squeezing, from one nipple only. If you notice any new lump that remains unchanged through one or two menstrual cycles, go and see your doctor. The vast majority of lumps detected through self-examination are not cancerous but they should always be checked by your doctor.

…ie down in a relaxed position …ith one hand behind your …ead and using the opposite …and feel round your breasts …ith your fingertips to check …r any unusual lumps.

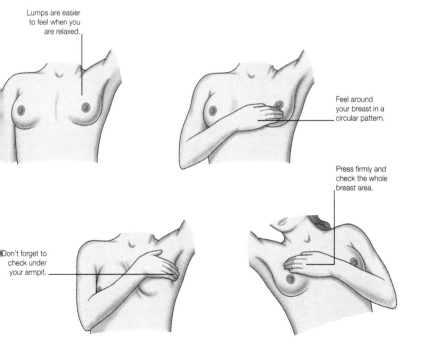

Lumps are easier to feel when you are relaxed.

Feel around your breast in a circular pattern.

Press firmly and check the whole breast area.

Don't forget to check under your armpit.

**I have heard that
too much circulating
oestrogen in the
body can cause
breast lumps and
cysts. Is this true?**

Both of the hormones oestrogen and progesterone have an effect on the breasts, which is why women often feel changes there before and after a period. Breast tissue changes during a woman's entire lifetime and is particularly sensitive to oestrogen and progesterone levels, which tend to fluctuate during the menstrual cycle. Changes in the hormone balance during normal, monthly menstrual cycles can create symptoms called fibrocystic changes. These are tiny, fluid-filled sacs that may feel like lumps. Tenderness and lump size commonly increase the week before your menstrual period and lessen a week after it. The lumps may be hard or rubbery, or may appear as a single breast lump, which can be either large or small.

Fibrocystic changes can occur in one or both breasts and are more common during your forties. They normally ease off during the menopause because there is less hormonal stimulation of the breast tissue. Some women also get breast cysts (*see Q 72*), which are fluid-filled sacs (usually benign) and are normally found in both breasts.

Fibroadenomas are the most common benign lumps. They are solid, round, rubbery lumps that move freely in the breast. Most common between the ages of 20 and 30, they are caused by an excess of milk-producing glands and connective tissue.

Intraductal papillomas are small, wart-like growths in the lining of the mammary duct near the nipple. They usually affect women of 45–50 years of age and can produce bleeding from the nipple. Traumatic fat necrosis occurs when there is trauma (sudden injury) to the breast that causes fat to form in lumps. These lumps are usually round, firm, hard, single and painless.

Occasionally breast lumps can indicate infection. Mastitis can occur in women who are breastfeeding and is caused by bacteria that enter the mammary ducts through the nipple. Localized infection will appear as tender, hot lumps in the breast (*see Q 40*).

My teenage daughter has just confided in me that she has one breast bigger than the other. I have told her that this is quite a normal development and that many women experience the same thing. Is this right?

Having one breast bigger than the other is extremely common, so reassure your teenager that she is not alone. In cases where one breast is larger than the other, it is more often the left one that is bigger. In theory, different breast size does not matter at all, as it has absolutely no bearing on a woman's sexuality or on her ability to breastfeed her babies. However, it can be hard to convince a teenager that breasts come in all sorts of different shapes and sizes and that hers fall within this normal range. The difference may not be obvious to anyone but your daughter, although if it is very marked, surgery to make the larger breast smaller (or vice versa) may be performed.

Q

16 **I have noticed that one of my nipples has started to discharge some fluid. What does this mean, and should I see my doctor?**

Nipple discharge is frightening for any woman, although two-thirds of women who are not pregnant can produce fluid simply by cleaning and massaging the breast. All women have fluid inside their breasts, but it does not normally find its way to the outside because the milk ducts are blocked with plugs of a substance called keratin.

During exercise or sexual activity the plug may become dislodged and the breast then releases a fluid, ranging from white through pale yellow to green or bluish black in colour. One of the most common forms of discharge occurs after childbirth, looks milky and continues to leak from the breast long after a woman has finished feeding her baby.

Some discharges are caused by duct disease, but a yellow or blood-stained discharge is most likely to be caused by a wart or papilloma in one of the ducts under the nipple. The duct can be removed surgically, after which the discharge usually stops.

Older women sometimes notice a thicker, cheesier discharge, and some women contract eczema on the skin around the nipple. This can be cured with a steroidal cream. In rare cases a form of breast cancer known as Paget's disease can also cause a discharge. Although a discharge is not normally a cause for concern, it is always worth seeing your doctor for your own peace of mind.

NIPPLE DISCHARGE

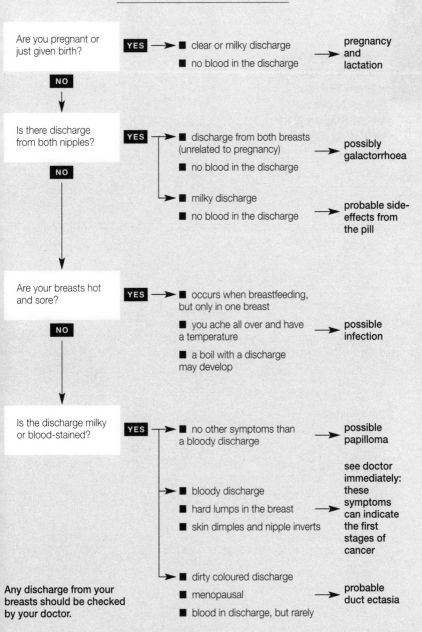

Are you pregnant or just given birth?

YES →
- clear or milky discharge
- no blood in the discharge

→ **pregnancy and lactation**

NO

Is there discharge from both nipples?

YES →
- discharge from both breasts (unrelated to pregnancy)
- no blood in the discharge

→ **possibly galactorrhoea**

- milky discharge
- no blood in the discharge

→ **probable side-effects from the pill**

NO

Are your breasts hot and sore?

YES →
- occurs when breastfeeding, but only in one breast
- you ache all over and have a temperature
- a boil with a discharge may develop

→ **possible infection**

NO

Is the discharge milky or blood-stained?

YES →
- no other symptoms than a bloody discharge

→ **possible papilloma**

- bloody discharge
- hard lumps in the breast
- skin dimples and nipple inverts

→ **see doctor immediately: these symptoms can indicate the first stages of cancer**

- dirty coloured discharge
- menopausal
- blood in discharge, but rarely

→ **probable duct ectasia**

Any discharge from your breasts should be checked by your doctor.

[37]

I have read that what you eat can affect your chances of getting cancer. Is there a dietary link with breast cancer?

The effect of the food we eat on our chances of getting breast cancer has been widely discussed, but it is difficult to draw any firm conclusions. In general, observational studies have shown that a low-fat, high-fibre diet with lots of antioxidants and green leafy vegetables lowers your risk of developing cancer, and at least five servings of fruit and vegetables a day are therefore recommended. And because breast cancer occurs in the UK at least six times as frequently as it does in Japan, some experts have theorized that eating soya products will also help. Again, the link has not been scientifically proven, but soya is known to have mild oestrogen-blocking effects and may be most helpful if it is eaten regularly before puberty.

In addition, dietary fat is a significant concern to women, when it comes to the risk of contracting breast cancer. In an analysis of fat samples drawn from the buttocks of 700 European women, researchers found that those with higher levels of trans fats had a 40 per cent greater risk of getting breast cancer. Trans fats are unsaturated fatty acids formed when vegetable oils are processed and are made more solid, or into a more stable liquid, by means of a process known as hydrogenation. Trans fats are present in variable amounts in a wide range of foods, including most foods made with partially hydrogenated oils, such as baked goods and fried foods, and in some margarine products. Trans fat is believed to make up as much as 10 per cent of the calories in a typical UK diet.

Researchers also found that women who reported eating few polyunsaturated fats, together with a high intake of trans fats, had three and a half times the risk of developing breast cancer, compared to women with a diet high in polyunsaturated fats (found in fish, vegetable oils and corn oils). Unfortunately, reducing your trans-fat intake does not bring an immediate drop in the risk for breast cancer. According to researchers, it takes a year or more to clear trans fat from stored body fat.

Is there any truth in the newspaper stories that if you have had breast implants you should never travel in a plane?

The story of a woman's breast implants exploding on a transatlantic flight is something of an urban myth and there is no evidence of it actually happening. It is probably based on the fact that early breast implants were prone to rupture. This can still happen with implants today – but less commonly, and it usually involves gentle seepage rather than a sudden explosion.

Ruptures are caused by tiny flaws in the silicone shell or by inadvertent needle pricks while the incision is being stitched up. It can also occur after a needle insertion (for a biopsy, for example) or when the breast is squeezed or compressed too tightly.

This can happen during procedures to break up fibrous tissue (capsular contracture) around the implant (see Q 62), or from a trauma, such as that caused by a car accident – or even, it is said, by an overenthusiastic hug. It is probably this pressure theory that led to the exploding-implant story! Rest assured that if you have breast implants, it is perfectly safe for you to fly.

Q 19

I read recently that scientists will soon be able to grow breasts from a woman's own body tissue. This sounds like the stuff of science fiction, not something that could be a reality within my own lifetime?

It is true that scientists have successfully carried out the first human trials of replacement nipples that have been grown in a laboratory. Although it is intended to develop the rest of the breasts using cells from a woman's own body, the nipples have in fact been constructed from cartilage derived from purified pig-ear cells.

Demand is expected to soar when natural tissue expansion can be used to enlarge breasts, instead of controversial artificial products such as silicone implants (see Q 62).

The tissue is grown using immature fat cells from elsewhere on a woman's body and is expanded in a laboratory on a frame of biodegradable 'scaffolding'. The expanded cell mass is then injected back into the breast. At present scientists are still searching for a material that is compatible with the body, which the host tissue can grow and then maintain in a natural-shaped breast.

I received an e-mail recently telling me that antiperspirants can cause breast cancer. Is this true?

This is a fine example of faulty cause-and-effect reasoning and came about as the result of a theory that antiperspirants prevent the body from sweating out toxins through the armpits. As most breast cancers are detected close to this area, people took this to its illogical conclusion – that is, that if there were more toxins in this area, then there must be a link to breast cancer.

The idea that your body could relegate the business of purging toxins to a few small skin areas is ludicrous, and there is no evidence to support this theory. What *is* true is that antiperspirants can interfere with the image produced by radiographic scanners so you are always told not to use one on the day that you have a mammogram.

There is also some truth in the theory that most breast cancers occur in the upper outer quadrant of the breast, but this is because most breast tissue is located here, and not because toxins have been unsuccessfully purged from the area.

Pregnancy &
Breastfeeding

Pregnancy and breastfeeding are two of the main times when a woman's breasts undergo radical changes in their appearance. For the first time in your life your breasts are fulfilling their primary biological function. Understanding the reasons for these changes may help you to cope with the alterations in your body and enable you to decide whether or not you wish to breast- or bottle-feed your baby.

Q

21

As my pregnancy progresses my breasts are getting really big, and a friend has said that I've got stretch marks on them. What exactly are stretch marks, and will they go away after I've had the baby?

When the skin on your stomach, breasts and thighs is stretched during pregnancy, the area becomes discoloured and results in stretch marks. In severe cases these appear as livid, red lines, but when your body returns to normal they usually fade to silvery lines on the skin. All stretch marks fade with time, although they won't disappear completely.

There is no guaranteed method of avoiding stretch marks, but many mothers swear by liberally applying vitamin E moisturizing creams, olive oil and moisturizing lotions during pregnancy.

I have only just found out that I'm pregnant, but my breasts are very tender and sore to the touch. Is this okay?

Soreness or tingling in your breasts during the early stages of pregnancy is common. You may also notice that your breasts get larger after about the eighth week and may seem lumpy or nodular. These are normal changes during pregnancy but you will find that taking a comfortably hot bath can provide welcome relief for sore breasts.

As your pregnancy progresses and your breasts feel heavier and more tender, you should buy a bra that will support you well, as this will help to ease any discomfort. Choose a bra (preferably of cotton) with a deep band under the cups, broad shoulder straps and an adjustable back. You should check your bra size regularly, as your breasts will continue to swell throughout pregnancy. By the time you are full-term you may have increased your cup measurement by up to two sizes. If your breasts become very heavy and uncomfortable you may want to wear a lightweight bra in bed at night.

23 I'm in the second
trimester of my
pregnancy and I've
noticed that the area
around my nipples is
getting darker. Is this
a cause for concern?

No, this is perfectly normal. The area surrounding the nipple, known as the areola, is normally pink before pregnancy, but turns brown or red-brown and may become larger during pregnancy and while you are breastfeeding. The areola may also produce little bumps called Montgomery's tubercules, which produce the necessary secretions to help prepare the nipples and areola for breastfeeding. These bumps are quite harmless and should not give you any cause for concern. However, on no account should you squeeze them or try to get secretions from them.

The darkening of the nipple and surrounding area that you will experience at around the 20-week mark may be accompanied by the appearance of a dark line (linea nigra) running down the centre of your stomach. This fades soon after the birth, although it may not disappear completely. As your pregnancy progresses you will probably notice that the veins on your breasts are more pronounced, too. These will also disappear when you stop breastfeeding. ●

I'm only about halfway through my pregnancy, but my breasts are discharging a liquid. Isn't it a bit early to be producing milk?

It is during pregnancy that we first come to realize the importance of our breasts. They are designed to secrete suitable nourishment for the baby during its first few months of life. The nine months of pregnancy not only allows the baby to prepare for life, but allows a woman's body to prepare for motherhood. The secretion you are experiencing at the moment is one of the natural stages your breasts go through during this preparation. It is not actually milk, but after the third month your breasts produce a cloudy yellow fluid called colostrum. Occasionally this leaks from the breasts or can be expressed by squeezing the nipples. This leakage is quite normal, but you should not try to express the fluid. It is best to invest in some breast pads if you have any problems or concerns.

Colostrum is a protein-rich food usually secreted by the breasts in the first days after the birth, and it supplies your baby with valuable antibodies against infection. This is replaced on around the fourth day by your milk supply, at which point the baby's sucking will stimulate your body into producing a plentiful supply.

I have very small
breasts, but I want
to breastfeed my
newborn baby and
am worried that I
won't have enough
milk to satisfy her?

The size of your breasts does not influence the amount of milk that you produce, and women with small breasts can breastfeed their baby just as successfully as full-breasted women. Regardless of size each breast contains enough of the milk producing glands to satisfy most babies appetites. The key to a good milk supply is not governed by breast size, but by feeding your baby when she wants to be fed. This can mean feeds at two- or three-hourly intervals in the early days, but this generally settles down to a regular routine after a few weeks, of four to five feeds per 24-hour period.

Breast-milk production works on the principle of supply and demand: the more frequently your baby feeds and the more she takes, the more milk you will produce. Although it is tempting to supplement a hungry baby with bottles of formula milk, this will simply wreck the system. If your baby is filled up on the bottle, she won't be keen to suckle from you, your breasts won't get the stimulation they need and your milk supply will dry up. This is true whether you have small or large breasts.

Irrespective of your breast size, what you need to do to produce enough breast milk is feed on demand, eat a good, nutritious diet, drink plenty of fluids and rest as much as possible. Your baby's appetite will guarantee the rest.

I've had a breast-reduction operation. Will this affect my ability to breastfeed in the future?

Unfortunately very few women who have had a breast-reduction operation are subsequently able to breastfeed successfully. This is a consequence of the surgery, during which the nipples are separated from the underlying milk ducts. As a result, during late pregnancy, when the body begins to produce milk for the impending birth, the milk supply has nowhere to go and it gradually dries up. This process is sometimes helped along artificially with the use of hormone treatment.

Your surgeon should have pointed out this consequence of a breast-reduction operation to you before you agreed to surgery. Tragically, this serves to emphasize further the importance of choosing a good and reputable surgeon in the first instance and discussing the consequences of breast operations before undergoing surgery (see Q 46). Women who have breasts that are only slightly larger than normal should consider the disadvantages of breast reduction very carefully: the inability to breastfeed and lack of sensation in the nipples.

I know it is of no consolation to you but, interestingly enough, women who have breast-enlargement surgery are more likely to be able to breastfeed successfully than those undergoing breast reductions. This is because the nipple does not have to be resited in a breast augmentation operation.

27 I have inverted nipples. Can I still breastfeed, and is there anything I can do to help myself before my baby is born?

Some women have inverted nipples, which are nipples that are flat or that invert (retract) into the breast. If so, you may experience some difficulty with breastfeeding, although most health professionals say that it is possible to breastfeed, but takes determination. Ask your doctor, midwife or breastfeeding counsellor for advice.

If you decide to give it a go, there are devices that you can use to help prepare your breasts for feeding. During the last few weeks of pregnancy start wearing breast shells. These plastic shells are worn inside your bra and create slight pressure at the base of the nipple, which helps to draw the nipple out. Ask your doctor or midwife for more information. ●

28 I'm expecting my first baby and, although I'm only six months pregnant, I want to get myself sorted out, but my mother-in-law says it's too soon to buy a nursing bra. Why is she raining on my parade?

I'm afraid that, on this occasion, your mother-in-law is right. Whilst it is perfectly understandable that you would want to get everything ready for you and your child as early as possible you should not buy a nursing bra before the thirty-sixth week of pregnancy at the earliest.

If you do buy your bra too soon, you may buy a bra that you think will fit but more than likely it will end up being the wrong size. At this stage it is impossible to tell exactly what sized bra you will need when the time comes as the size of your breasts will fluctuate between pregnancy and breastfeeding.

Nursing bras are designed with cups that are detachable so that you can breastfeed without having to undress. Once the baby is born and your milk comes in, your breasts will become larger, so you should buy a nursing bra with at least a finger's width of space between the bra and your breast. You should also allow a little space for breast pads. When trying on a bra, fasten it at the loosest setting. In this way you can tighten it as your ribcage shrinks after the baby is born. You should buy your nursing bra as near to your due date as possible.

My breasts have grown a lot during my pregnancy. Will they return to their normal size after breastfeeding?

When you stop breastfeeding your breasts should return to their normal size, although some women find that, if anything, their breasts are slightly smaller after breastfeeding. This is because milk glands have replaced some of the fatty tissue, and the connective tissue that forms the support system in the breasts has changed.

Exercise cannot make breasts any firmer, but it can improve the musculature in the chest area so that your breasts get better support, which in turn makes them look perter. It is a fallacy that breastfeeding makes your breasts droop. Sadly, it is time, gravity and weight gain that are responsible for the sagging process.

30 Due to work
and domestic
commitments I
have been unable
to attend antenatal
classes. I feel that
I'd like to breastfeed
my baby, but I don't
know where to start.
Will the baby know
what to do, or will
I need some
instruction?

To an extent it's true that breastfeeding is instinctive for both mother and baby. However, it is probably fair to say that it doesn't come naturally to many new mothers and that you may have an easier time if you have some understanding of the principles involved.

Your baby will instinctively search for your nipple to find food – this is known as the rooting reflex. Until she is about ten days old you can stimulate this reflex by stroking the cheek nearest to your breast; she will automatically turn towards your breast and search for the nipple. If she doesn't respond in this way, try gently squeezing a few drops of milk from your nipple and touching her lips to it, to encourage her to feed. As she opens her mouth, bring her head up close to your breast, so that her chin rests against it and her tongue is just underneath your nipple. Then guide your breast into her mouth.

This is called 'latching-on', and your baby should open her jaws wide and take the whole of the nipple and most of the surrounding areola into her mouth in order to latch on successfully. When she starts to feed, your baby's jaws will 'milk' the breast by rhythmically pressing on the reservoirs of milk at the base of the areola. Breathe deeply as she starts to feed in order to relax yourself. If you are in any doubt as to whether or not she has latched on

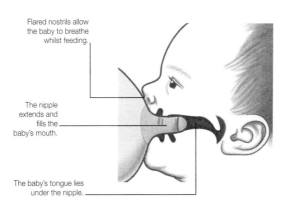

Flared nostrils allow the baby to breathe whilst feeding.

The nipple extends and fills the baby's mouth.

The baby's tongue lies under the nipple.

Breastfeeding does not involve your baby sucking on a nipple, she milks the breast by pressing her jaws on the reservoirs of milk at the base of the areola.

properly, look at her temples and ears. If they are moving rhythmically, then her jaw muscles are working hard and she has probably latched on properly. If your baby just sucks at the nipple, you will get sore very quickly and she won't get enough milk to satisfy her.

Although you have missed antenatal classes you may still benefit from getting in touch with a breastfeeding counsellor. Your midwife may well be able to give you good advice, or a counsellor from the international La Lèche Society or from the National Childbirth Trust in the UK (*see page 138*) will definitely be able to help. Once you have got the hang of breastfeeding over the first week or so, it is entirely up to you how long you continue to breastfeed, but this can be a very special, close and satisfying experience for both you and your baby.

Q

31 My friend said that she froze breast milk for her baby. Surely this can't be right? Wouldn't frozen milk harm the baby?

It may come as a surprise, but you can freeze expressed breast milk for up to six months in a deep-freeze (at -29°C/-20°F). Store the milk in a sterilized, sealed bottle in small quantities, because these are easier to thaw quickly. When required, it can then be thawed at room temperature for at least four hours (never microwave breast milk, as this can alter the composition of the milk), ready for someone else to give to your baby while you are out. You can also store breast milk safely in the refrigerator for up to 72 hours.

Some mothers express their milk by hand. This involves systematically massaging each breast, working down and around the breast towards the areola to stimulate the flow of milk through the ducts.

After about ten circuits, press gently on the area behind the areola with your thumbs and fingers and, while squeezing gently and pulling back from the nipple,

Supporting your breast massage working down from above the breast.

Work around the breast, including the underside to help the milk flow through the ducts.

Use your fingertips to stroke downwards to the areola.

Apply gentle pressure with thumb and finger behind the areola. Milk should come out of the nipple.

Expressing milk by hand is easy and painless. Make sure you are relaxed, apply warm towels to your breasts to help the milk flow, and make sure your bowl is sterilized.

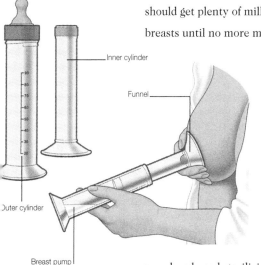

Expressing milk by pump may be more painful than by hand, but it is quicker. Make sure that all the equipment is sterilized, and apply warm towels to your breast to ease the milk flow.

Inner cylinder

Funnel

Outer cylinder

Breast pump

the milk should start to flow. Continue for a few minutes and then repeat the massaging action on the other breast. After squeezing out a little milk, return to the original breast and repeat the procedure. By now the milk flow should be established and you should get plenty of milk. Alternate between the breasts until no more milk flows. Most women who express by hand recommend having a warm bath or placing warm flannels on the breasts before you start both to relax you and to help the milk flow. Make sure that you are as clean as possible before you start by washing your hands and sterilizing the bowl into which you are expressing.

If all this sounds too much hard work, then you might want to try using a pump. You can get a 'syringe'-style hand pump or an electric pump. The funnel needs to cover the areola and form an airtight seal – the pressure works the milk ducts, just as your baby's jaws would do. Some mothers report that these 'contraptions' are more painful than hand-expressing but, once you get the hang of things, they are certainly faster and less tiring. You will find that the tip of softening the breasts in warm water before expressing works just as well with this method.

32 I have to go back to
work when my baby
is three and a half
months old, but I
want to continue
to breastfeed her
throughout the first
year. What can I do?

Many mothers successfully manage to combine
returning to work with continuing to
breastfeed. In order to keep your milk supply
stimulated, you will need to express milk at the
times you would normally feed your baby. This takes
some planning, but, if you stick to the following
guidelines, you should be able to breastfeed your
baby indefinitely.

First, you need to be confident that your baby will
accept milk from a bottle, so ask your partner or a
friend to introduce her to her first bottle-feeds before
you return to work. If you try yourself, she will smell
your breast milk and refuse the bottle. Leave bottles
of expressed milk for your baby's daytime feeds. In
the meantime, make sure that you have somewhere
private at work to express milk during the day, and a
fridge to store it in until you go home. A small
freezer bag with ice packs is ideal for transporting
your expressed milk. Also, ask your baby-carer to
delay the teatime feed so you can breastfeed on your
return. Some women prefer to drop the daytime
expressing and simply breastfeed at night and in the
morning – expressing during the evening in order to
leave bottles for the next day.

Although you can breastfeed well into your baby's
second year if you are both still happy with it, most
women cease breastfeeding during the latter half of

their baby's first year. You may even find that your baby gives up the daytime feeds of her own accord at around the nine-month mark. When you want to give up breastfeeding you should let your milk supply dry up slowly over an extended period. Drop one feed at a time (usually the midday feed first), leaving at least three days before dropping another feed. You will experience a 'full' feeling for the first day or so, but the milk is gradually reabsorbed over a few days and the feeling will pass. Don't be tempted to express or you will simply perpetuate the full feeling.

The last feed to drop is the night-feed. Most babies are comforted by sucking, so you may want to replace this feed with a bottle or beaker at bedtime. Breast or formula milk should be used for the first year, but cow's milk is safe thereafter.

3 **My baby bites me when she is feeding and it really hurts. How can I stop her?**

If your baby bites you whilst feeding, take her off the breast straight away, with a stern look; you can even say 'no' very loudly. Repeat this procedure every time she bites and she will soon get the message that this is unacceptable behaviour. Many babies will attempt to bite a nursing mother once, but it is not malicious and is not sufficient reason to give up feeding. Most babies only need to be told off sharply once and they won't repeat this behaviour. If she persists, then you may decide that it is time to call it a day.

My baby always seems hungry and I'm not sure that I'm making enough milk for her. How can I tell?

The vast majority of women do produce enough milk to satisfy their babies. Trust your baby to know how much she wants and needs at any given time. She will let you know when she's had enough. Usually, once her appetite is sated, she will fall fast asleep in your arms and let your nipple slip from her mouth. As long as your baby's weight is increasing steadily there should be no cause for concern. If you are worried you can discuss this with your midwife or your doctor.

Breast milk is not the same throughout the feed. At the beginning, your baby takes fore-milk, which is watery and thirst-quenching. Then she gets to the hind-milk, which is rich in calories and more satisfying. In order to ensure that your baby gets all the nutrients she needs you should allow her to suck for at least 10–15 minutes on one breast at each feed, or she will soon wake up hungry again.

However, it is fair to say that a few mothers do find that their baby is still hungry after a feed. Sometimes you don't have enough milk because of dehydration or deficiencies in your diet, or simply because you are exhausted. To try and prevent or counteract this situation, make sure that during the day you drink at least 3 litres of water and that you are eating a fully balanced nutritional diet. Many health professionals recommend that you should also have a glass of water or juice next to you to drink while you breastfeed. You should also make sure that you are getting a well-balanced diet; you may even consider taking suitable supplements, but consult your doctor or complementary medical practitioner before taking anything.

Finally, difficult though it may be to achieve, try and get as much sleep and rest as possible. All these measures will help with your milk production.

Is it true that, if I breastfeed, my nipples will drip milk whenever my baby cries? My friend told me this, but I think she's just winding me up.

I have to tell you that this is no wind-up. Whenever your baby or another baby near you cries, it triggers a reflex known as the 'milk let-down response', and this in turn activates your milk production. It is a perfectly normal reaction, if a little embarrassing on occasions.

The let-down reflex is usually triggered by your baby's sucking action, but it can also be sparked off by crying, and unfortunately your body cannot distinguish between the cries of babies. So remember to wear breast pads to absorb any drips and to protect your clothing. However, you must change the pads frequently, as wetness near your skin can make you sore. If you leak a lot, try using a plastic breast shell (see Q 36).

36 I am breastfeeding at the moment and my breasts often leak at just the wrong moment. What can I do to prevent this?

If you are concerned about embarrassing leaks, you should wear breast shells. These are plastic 'cups' that separate into two halves, with a hole in one side for the nipple, and they collect any milk that may leak, without marking your clothes. They are also useful if you have sore nipples because they allow air to circulate around the nipples, so letting them dry naturally, which prevents cracking. The expressed milk that you collect in the breast shells can be poured into a sterile bottle and refrigerated or frozen (*see Q 31*) for later use. Make sure that you wash and sterilize the breast shells before reusing them.

From personal experience, I would just add that you should try to remember to empty breast shells regularly and watch out if you bend over – if you haven't emptied them recently, the milk can spill out, with disastrous effects.

If you are simply experiencing a slightly damp patch rather than full-blown leakage, you could simply wear breast pads inside your nursing bra. Remember to change these regularly since it is often the friction of your nipples against damp material that causes sore and cracked nipples. ●

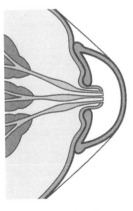

Breast shells are domed-shaped plastic containers that fit inside your nursing bra to catch any milk leakages.

I get a strange, tingling sensation in my breasts when my baby starts to nurse. What causes this?

When a woman first starts to breastfeed her baby, many experience a tingling or mild cramping sensation in their breast. This is a perfectly normal reaction and nothing to be concerned about. This sensation that you are experiencing is called the 'milk let-down response' and it signals that the milk is beginning to flow into the ducts in your nipples.

Your baby's sucking action stimulates your breasts to release the milk they have stored. The tingling sensation is caused as you feel the warm rush of milk coming through. It usually happens at the beginning of a feed and several times throughout. Sometimes your baby can choke slightly if the surge of milk comes too quickly. Just sit her up until she has caught her breath, then latch her on again. However, not everyone feels the let-down reflex, so don't worry or be surprised if you don't. If the reflex causes the other breast to leak milk too, hold a breast pad over your nipple to catch the drips or use a breast shell. Some women report that this reaction can sometimes be triggered when they hear their baby, or indeed any baby, crying. It is a response to your baby's hunger signals (*see Q 35*).

My milk has just come in and my breasts are completely engorged and very tender. I'm so depressed by the pain that I am tempted to give up breastfeeding and start with a bottle. Is there anything I can do to relieve the pressure, or shall I just give up?

For the first few days after the birth your baby feeds on a yellow fluid called colostrum (*see Q 24*). Between two and six days after the birth your breasts start to produce mature milk, rather than colostrum, and you may well wake up to find your breasts swollen, hard and uncomfortable. This is commonly known as engorgement, and it may cause you some pain or discomfort usually only for a day or so.

Apart from being uncomfortable for you, when your breasts are engorged your baby will find it hard to latch onto the breast to feed, because the nipple is flattened out by the swollen areola. To help you get through this difficult early stage you can soften your breasts by laying warm flannels over them for several minutes before feeding your baby. Alternatively, you can stand in the shower and splash warm water over your breasts or soak them in a bowl of warm water. Gently massaging your breasts with your hands to

When your milk comes in, about the fourth day of breastfeeding, the areola becomes swollen and the nipple flattened and uncomfortable. This may last for a couple of days but will be relieved when you feed your baby.

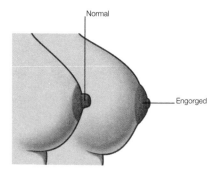

Normal

Engorged

express some of the milk can also help to relieve the swelling, thus making your breasts less painful and easier for your baby to latch onto. Once successfully latched on, her sucking will quickly relieve the engorgement and discomfort. Although it is painful and discouraging to have engorged breasts, try to persevere during this time because once through these difficult few days, breastfeeding becomes not only much easier and less uncomfortable but a worthwhile experience for both you and your baby.

While your breasts are engorged you should wear a nursing bra for support; a cool cabbage leaf from the fridge placed inside your bra is a wonderful old wives' tale that really works – it gives remarkable relief. If the hot flannel treatment or warm bath treatments don't work, some mothers swear by cold compresses, but use these for brief periods only. If the pain is severe, take paracetamol after the baby's feed, so that your body can metabolize it before the baby's next meal; if the swelling and discomfort persist, consult your doctor or midwife.

The homeopathic remedies Phytolacca 6 or Natrum muriaticum 6, taken every quarter of an hour, may help. Some mothers who have suffered with recurrent engorgement problems recommend acupuncture and herbal treatment as highly beneficial. The supplements vitamin B_6, evening primrose oil and zinc are all helpful in reducing breast fluid retention – a feature of engorgement – and do not affect the baby's breast milk.

BREASTFEEDING PROBLEMS

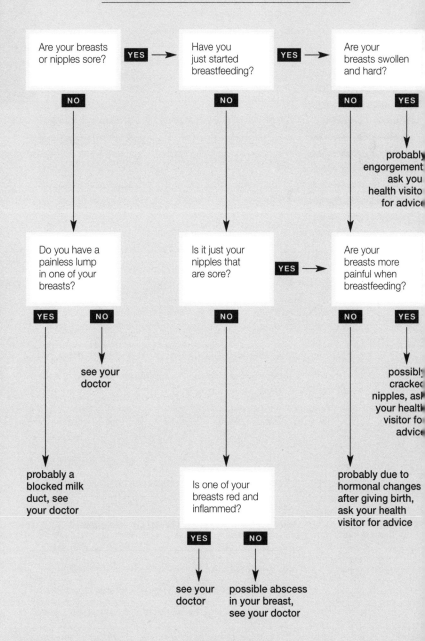

Are your breasts or nipples sore? → **YES** → Have you just started breastfeeding? → **YES** → Are your breasts swollen and hard?

Are your breasts swollen and hard? **YES** → probably engorgement ask you health visito for advice

Are your breasts or nipples sore? **NO** → Do you have a painless lump in one of your breasts?

Do you have a painless lump in one of your breasts? **YES** → probably a blocked milk duct, see your doctor

Do you have a painless lump in one of your breasts? **NO** → see your doctor

Have you just started breastfeeding? **NO** → Is it just your nipples that are sore? **YES** → Are your breasts more painful when breastfeeding?

Are your breasts swollen and hard? **NO** → Are your breasts more painful when breastfeeding?

Are your breasts more painful when breastfeeding? **YES** → possibl cracked nipples, as your health visitor fo advice

Are your breasts more painful when breastfeeding? **NO** → probably due to hormonal changes after giving birth, ask your health visitor for advice

Is it just your nipples that are sore? **NO** → Is one of your breasts red and inflamed?

Is one of your breasts red and inflamed? **YES** → see your doctor

Is one of your breasts red and inflamed? **NO** → possible abscess in your breast, see your doctor

[62]

I'm expecting my second baby and I had a miserable time with my first, because I suffered terribly from cracked and bleeding nipples. Is there any way to prevent sore nipples when breastfeeding, because I don't want to go through the same experience with my second baby?

The major cause of sore nipples is due to the baby not latching onto the breast properly. For new mums, in particular, it is such a blessed relief that the baby is feeding at all that we are reluctant to start all over again if they don't appear to be latched on correctly. However, this is a mistake. It is so important to make sure that your baby is latching onto the breast correctly when she feeds (*see Q 30*). If she doesn't take all of the nipple and part of the areola into her mouth fully during feeding, then her gums will end up gnawing on your nipple and this will make you very sore. If she doesn't latch on properly, gently take her off the breast and start again. Do this by carefully slipping a finger between her jaws to break the suction – if you pull your nipple away abruptly, it will hurt you.

Sore nipples rarely last more than a few days, but it is miserable and painful while the condition lasts. So the best advice is to try to continue to breastfeed during this time, but in between feeds, try wearing a nipple shield to provide some relief. This plastic device is worn inside the bra and stops the nipple from rubbing against the bra fabric; it also allows air to circulate around the nipple, which is beneficial. To prevent sore nipples, it is advisable to dry your nipples after each feed – some mothers recommend a hair-drier on a cool setting for maximum comfort.

In addition, once your baby has emptied the milk from your breast, don't allow her to continue sucking. Let the air get to your nipples often, and wash them with water, not soap (which dries the skin). Dry them well. You can also change the position in which your baby feeds to alter the pressure points on the nipple and areola and this can prevent sore pressure points from forming.

If none of this works and you are blighted with sore nipples, you'll find that a mild calendula-based cream or antiseptic spray can provide welcome relief. Always ask your pharmacist or doctor about suitable products before applying anything to the nipples while nursing.

If your nipples are giving you severe pain, you can express milk from the most uncomfortable breast for a day or so rather than directly. This will give your tender nipple a chance to recover. If your nipple is cracked, giving you a shooting pain each time the baby sucks, try a 'sombrero' shield. This is placed over the nipple before you put your baby to the breast, and she sucks milk through it. Sterilize it well before use and rub it with a drop of breast milk to disguise the rubbery smell. You could also try the homeopathic remedy Graphite or Silica (potency 6) which are both recommended for cracked nipples, but again you should discuss this with your doctor, midwife or health visitor before using it.

Occasionally a milk duct in the breast gets plugged, thereby preventing the milk from flowing freely. This results in a tender or firm area on the breast that becomes more painful after breastfeeding. If you continue to nurse frequently, this problem usually sorts itself out. You can apply warm compresses to the sore area or soak the breast in warm water to help with the pain and to open the duct. Gentle massage may also help.

However, occasionally a blocked milk duct may become infected, causing a flu-like fever to develop. The first signs of a breast infection (mastitis) are large red streaks extending up the breast towards the armpit, accompanied by breast pain. An infection may cause a fever to develop within four to eight hours of the first appearance of these streaks, in which case you should call your doctor without

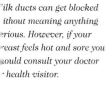

ilk ducts can get blocked ithout meaning anything rious. However, if your reast feels hot and sore you ould consult your doctor health visitor.

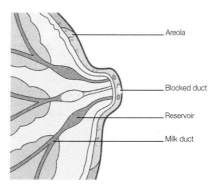

Areola

Blocked duct

Reservoir

Milk duct

delay. You will be prescribed a course of antibiotics (which it is imperative that you complete) and, if you catch the infection early enough, this treatment should clear up the infection within 24 hours. You can continue to breastfeed if you are taking antibiotics, as long as you know the drug is not incompatible with nursing, but you may also need to rest in bed and empty the infected breast by expressing or breastfeeding every hour or two.

Self-help treatments for breast infection include: applying hot and cold compresses to the area; putting cabbage leaves from the fridge or freezer over the inflammation; and gently massaging the area with a cream containing arnica. If a breast infection is left untreated, it may lead to a breast abscess, which is not only excruciatingly painful but may need surgery to open and drain it.

Of course, prevention is better than cure and there are several things you can do to help prevent a blocked duct or infection, including: making sure that your nursing bra is not too tight; eating correctly and getting enough rest; taking care not to press too hard on the breast tissue when you feed or express; and ensuring that you empty your breasts regularly, as this avoids engorgement.

A friend told me that breastfeeding may prevent milk allergies. Is this true?

It is nearly impossible for a baby to become allergic to its mother's milk. So the longer a baby breastfeeds, the less likely she is to be exposed to substances that could cause allergic problems.

Breast milk also contains high levels of immunoglobulins, which are part of the baby's first line of defence against infection. Eczema, asthma and hay fever are less common in breastfed babies and, since colic is often associated with an allergic response, it is believed that breastfed babies may suffer less from this, too.

If you have any history of allergy in your family, then it would be desirable to breastfeed your baby if at all possible. This will not necessarily prevent your child from getting allergies, but it may lessen the probability or the severity of an attack.

We've got a wedding four weeks after my baby's due. I want to wear a tight-fitting suit that I bought before I found out I was pregnant and I've been told not to diet while breast-feeding. Is this true?

Yes, it is best not to diet while breastfeeding. The nutrients your baby receives while breastfeeding are totally dependent on the quality of the food you eat and there are actually more demands on your body during breastfeeding than during pregnancy. You burn up to 1000 calories a day just producing enough milk to feed your baby, so while breastfeeding you need to eat an extra 500 calories a day and be sure to keep your fluid levels up. Eat when you are hungry and make sure that you get your calories from fresh, vitamin-rich food rather than the 'empty' calories in snacks or junk foods.

Don't worry too much about getting back to your pre-pregnancy size. You actually gain your figure more quickly if you breastfeed, because the hormones released encourage the uterus to shrink back to normal quite fast; the fat reserves that your body lays down during pregnancy are used in the production of breast milk; and your waistline contracts sooner, too.

Nonetheless, many women expect to feel thinner as soon as they have delivered. However, although you lose on average 4.5–6.75kg (10–15lb) immediately after your baby is born, the remaining weight may be harder to shift. Your body stores around 3.15–4.5kg (7–10lb) of fat to provide energy for the first few months after the birth. If you eat healthily and get enough exercise, these extra pounds should come off.

On a cautionary note, be careful about beginning an exercise programme too soon. Discuss it with your doctor before you start and take it slowly. Walking and swimming are excellent ways to help.

Even if you do manage to get back into shape in time to slip into your slinky outfit for the family wedding, you can expect to have a larger bust if you are still breastfeeding, which may or may not enhance the look.

I find the whole idea of breastfeeding quite repulsive, so I've decided that I don't even want to try to breastfeed my newborn. Can I have an injection or pills to dry up my milk, or will it have to happen naturally? And what if I change my mind and decide that I want to breastfeed later on?

If you know categorically that you do not want to breastfeed, you may be given pills to stop your milk supply from coming in, but this practice is becoming less and less common. More often now your breasts will be bound or wrapped to stop the milk flow.

Whether to breast- or bottle-feed your baby is a very personal decision, and whatever you decide is fine. If you want to bottle-feed, you should not be made to feel guilty in any way – there are distinct advantages and disadvantages to both methods. However, if it is a preference rather than a definite decision, then it may be a good idea to put off finally choosing until after the baby is born. The colostrum that your breasts produce in the first few days will provide your baby with valuable antibodies to help fight infection in her early months.

Once you have started bottle-feeding, you can't switch back to breastfeeding because, without the stimulation of your baby's sucking, your breasts will stop producing milk. In that sense, it is a very final decision, so you must be sure in your own mind that you definitely do not want to breastfeed when you embark on a bottle-feeding programme.

Whatever your decision, remember that the love, attention and nurture you give to your baby are just as important as the type of milk you feed her.

44 **My mother says that breastfeeding is the best way to bond with your baby. Is this an old wives' tale?**

It is certainly true that breastfeeding is an excellent way to bond with your baby because of the physical closeness and the intimacy of the feeding process. It is also the case that at first babies can most easily focus on objects about 20cm/8in away. This means that breastfeeding gives them the best opportunity to study their mother's face which in turn aids recognition and bonding.

Many mothers report that they establish an early relationship with their baby because of the exclusive nature of this type of feeding. However, breastfeeding alone is no guarantee that you will immediately bond with your baby. You may well love your baby immediately, but if you don't feel instant love for your newborn that is not unusual, either. This bond will grow over time as you and your baby get to know each other.

The good news for human survival is that, irrespective of your feelings or the way you choose to feed your infant, a baby will instinctively seek out someone to protect her. From birth a baby will cling, cuddle, make eye contact and respond to an adult's efforts to soothe her – all responses designed to stimulate our bonding instincts. So even without breastfeeding bonding with your baby would be difficult to avoid.

A friend of mine has told me that I can't get pregnant while I'm breastfeeding. She said she used this method of contraception and it was perfectly safe. Is this true?

You cannot rely on breastfeeding to protect you against getting pregnant again. There is a grain of truth in what your friend says, in that your body produces hormones while you are breastfeeding that reduce your fertility, but you definitely need to use some type of contraceptive protection when you make love.

Routine oral contraceptives are not recommended if you are breastfeeding. Some doctors believe that the oral pill can reduce breast-milk production. It is also known that tiny traces of the hormones used in oral contraceptives can get into your breast milk and be passed on to your baby. Although it is unlikely that they can adversely affect your baby's development, not enough is known of their effects to take a chance. Some doctors will prescribe progestogen-only oral contraceptives to breastfeeding mothers, but most recommend that you use some form of barrier method of birth control until you have finished breastfeeding. Consult your doctor for detailed advice.

Cosmetic Surgery

The shape, size and appearance of a woman's breasts can be intrinsically linked to how she views herself as a woman. Many women feel that they can improve their appearance and self-esteem by altering the size and shape of their breasts using cosmetic surgery. Some women have very different reasons for considering surgery – those who lose one or both breasts because of breast cancer. This section discusses the implications of cosmetic breast surgery.

46 **I've made my mind up to have a breast increase. I don't know anyone who has had the operation and I don't want to ask my doctor for advice because he's a family friend. How can I find a surgeon who has specific training in my cosmetic breast-surgery procedure?**

It is really important that you think about your decision carefully before having any cosmetic operation on your breasts. There are consequences that you must consider, and you should discuss these fully with your surgeon before going ahead. In order to ensure that you are fully informed you must choose a surgeon who specializes in cosmetic breast surgery, and one in whom you feel confident.

Before committing to a specific specialist, ask how many procedures of this kind he or she has performed? And how many are currently being performed each year? Many surgeons have before-and-after photographs of previous patients and this can give you some indication of a surgeon's ability, although you cannot take these as any sort of guarantee concerning your own results, since each patient differs. You should also feel entirely comfortable with your chosen surgeon and at ease with the other staff. Make sure that your concerns are addressed to your satisfaction and that all your questions are answered fully. Most countries have a professional body governing cosmetic surgeons (for examples, *see page 141*), which will be able to provide a list of qualified surgeons.

What sort of credentials should I be looking for in a surgeon?

It is important to satisfy yourself that your surgeon is suitably qualified for the job, and board certification is one of the yardsticks that you can use in judging a surgeon's qualifications. Ask about his or her qualifications, who accredited these and study them carefully.

There are several professional societies (*see page 141*) to which surgeons may belong and some are more specialized – and more stringent in their requirements – than others, so you are best advised to check your doctor's society affiliation and then to call the society to find out what their requirements for membership are. As a general rule of thumb, most speciality boards require at least four years of residency training in plastic and/or cosmetic surgical procedures to provide a solid base for a surgeon's skills but some boards also ask for extra experience.

48

Q

I have very large breasts that cause me considerable pain and discomfort, not to mention the way in which they have negatively affected my confidence. Can I get cosmetic breast surgery done on my insurance?

Some women with very large breasts suffer from back, neck, breast and shoulder pain due to the weight of the breasts. They may also get grooves cut into their shoulders from bra straps and rashes under the bust from trapped sweat. Many women also report that the activities in which they can participate are limited because of discomfort (even running for a bus may be a painful experience). Many women find that because of the sexual nature of breasts, the prominence of a very large bust may attract unwanted attention from the opposite sex, ribald comments, sexual innuendoes and even unwanted advances.

Many large-breasted women confess that their appearance and the attention that it attracts, combined with the physical discomforts they suffer, can cause them considerable psychological and emotional distress.

Because of these adverse reactions, some insurance policies will often cover some or all of the costs of this type of surgery. However, do make sure that you check with your insurance provider before undergoing surgery. You can also ask the surgeon's secretary or the hospital administrators for advice.

My friend has a fear of hospitals, but she wants to have a breast-reduction operation. Will she need a full anaesthetic and a hospital stay if she goes ahead with cosmetic surgery, or can this be avoided?

A breast-reduction operation is fairly major surgery and an anaesthetic will generally be needed. In Britain your friend would probably have to stay in the hospital or clinic for several days after the operation. In the US, however, these procedures can be performed on an outpatient basis in the hospital, or in an ambulatory suite under either general or local anaesthesia as necessary.

If your friend decides that she cannot face the surgical procedure, there are ways to disguise a large bust, such as wearing a minimizer bra and dressing in looser-fitting shirts and tops. Choosing a well-fitted bra is even more important if you have a large bust (see Q 1), and it will actually make your bust look smaller if you get a properly fitted one rather than trying to squeeze into a smaller size.

Minimizing bras are designed to give added support and minimize size whilst retaining shape.

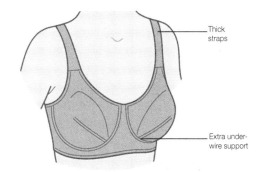

Thick straps

Extra under-wire support

Q

50 I am self-employed and cannot afford much time off work. I am thinking about having a breast lift. Can you tell me what recovery time is needed after this kind of operation?

A breast lift (or mastopexy, to use the technical term) is a fairly serious operation that requires a general anaesthetic. You will probably need just an overnight stay in hospital, depending on the extent of the procedure. However, you will have to refrain from strenuous physical exercise for a month afterwards and you will probably need at least two weeks off work (which can, of course, be something of a problem for the self-employed who do not get holiday pay). You should also bear in mind that if there are any complications with your surgery, then the time needed off work could stretch into weeks or even months.

Q

51 I'd like to have some breast implants, but a friend who had hers done said that it was a really painful process. Is she an exception, or is this generally true?

Most women experience some discomfort or mild pain after a breast-augmentation operation and you can expect a fair deal of swelling and bruising for several days after the surgery. Of course, each individual's tolerance to pain varies, but in the vast majority of cases the discomfort can easily be controlled with pain-relief medication. Perhaps your friend has a particularly low pain threshold or had minor complications with her surgical procedure that caused her additional pain and discomfort.

I am starting out on a modelling career and want to have a breast-augmentation operation to increase my employment prospects. However, as I will be modelling swimwear and underwear I am worried that the scars may show in the photographs. Will the scars be visible in skimpy clothing?

Depending on where your surgeon makes the incisions for your breast implants, you will always have scars on the breast or in the armpit. Each individual surgeon has his own preferred choice of incision site but all result in some scarring. The scars will settle over a period of 12 months or so, and their appearance varies considerably from individual to individual. For some, the scars are only very faint and scarcely noticeable, while for others the scarring is more defined.

In the majority of cases the scarring is minimal and it is placed in such a position that it is barely visible (if at all), even in a skimpy swimming costume. You should have no problems in pursuing a career in fashion modelling and I think you will find that there are many models who are successful because of rather than in spite of their breast-enlargement operations. Nonetheless, you should make sure that you explain your concerns to your surgeon before the operation, as this may affect his or her decision on where the incisions are made.

Q 53 I have very large and heavy breasts and I suffer from backache and neck pain as a result. My parents are prepared to pay for me to have a breast-reduction operation, but none of us knows what's involved. Can you explain?

In the most basic of terms, breast reduction involves the removal of excess fat and skin from the breasts, which are then reshaped and the nipples repositioned to form newer, smaller breasts. There are several different surgical designs to reshape the breasts, but all of them will involve a scar around the areola (the dark area surrounding the nipple). Each method will produce scars in different places, with its own advantages and disadvantages. With your approval, your surgeon will select the best technique for your particular case.

The operation is usually carried out under a general anaesthetic in the UK, although in the US a local anaesthetic may be used. When you awake after the operation you will experience some discomfort, which will last for two or three days. Don't worry, though – you will be given suitable pain-relief injections or tablets. Drainage tubes are frequently used and will be removed after a short

Mastopexy operations give uplift to droopy breasts. However, scars will be left (as shown) and because the nipples are moved it is unlikely that you would be able to breastfeed and many women report less sensation in the nipples during sexual intercourse.

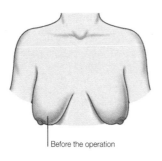
Before the operation

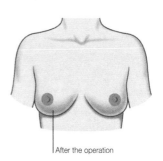
After the operation

period of time, but you will probably have to stay in hospital for three or four days in the UK, although in the US this may not be necessary.

The stitches are normally removed 10–14 days later and you should expect to feel tired enough to need some help around the home for a period of between two and six weeks, depending on your age and general fitness. You will need to wear a well-fitting bra following surgery but, because of the post-operative swelling and bruising, the final size of your breasts may not be apparent for several weeks. There is likely to be some tenderness and lumpiness in the breasts for several weeks – or even months – after the operation, but you are free to sunbathe and go swimming once the scars have fully healed.

If I have a breast-reduction mammoplasty operation, will I be scarred?

The scars from a breast-reduction operation are designed to be invisible when you are wearing normal clothing and, as far as possible, should lie under the average bra or bikini top.

Over the months following surgery the scars will fade from an angry red (and possibly a thick and uncomfortable appearance) to a much paler and less obvious colour. However, you should bear in mind that they will always be present and visible when you are completely undressed and that scarring will vary from individual to individual. Some women are lucky enough to have very thin white lines, while other women have an inborn tendency for scars to stretch and may end up with scars that are thick, red and irritable for quite some time. However, it has to be said that the vast majority of women who undergo a breast-reduction procedure would say that the scars are an acceptable trade-off for the benefits of not having to deal with the pain and unwanted attention caused by extremely large breasts.

After a breast reduction it is occasionally necessary to adjust the folds of skin at the end of the scar, both between the breasts and at the sides. This is a simple procedure and will most likely be carried out under local anaesthetic a couple of months after the initial operation. ●

55 **I'm going in for a breast-reduction operation in about three months' time. My doctor has recommended that I lose over 3kg/7lb in weight before the operation. Why is that, and is there anything else I should do to help ensure the success of the operation?**

Your surgeon has probably recommended that you reduce your weight because you are at less risk from the adverse effects of a general anaesthetic if you are not overweight.

You may also be advised to stop taking the contraceptive pill or to change to an alternative method at least six weeks before the operation. Smoking can seriously effect the healing of your breast wounds so, if possible, you should give up or cut down. Incidentally, this advice applies to any cosmetic breast-surgery procedure. ●

My sister has had a breast-reduction operation and says that she now gets less pleasure from sexual foreplay. Is this usual?

Your sister's experience is not exceptional. Because the nipple has to be cut and resited on the breast, this affects the nerve supply, so some women experience a numbness in the nipples that occasionally extends over part of the breast as well. This usually wears off with time, but the nipples are likely to be very much less sensitive following surgery. This diminished sensitivity probably accounts for your sister's reduced pleasure from sexual foreplay that involves her breasts.

I have had a breast reduction and am delighted with the results. I just feel so much more confident about my appearance, but now I'm frightened that the improvements won't last. Am I being silly?

I am assuming that you are of an age when your breasts have stopped growing (that is, post-puberty), so they should not regrow after a breast-reduction procedure. Indeed, the operation should not have been preformed on a pubescent girl. However, you should be aware that your breasts will increase in size if you either put on weight or become pregnant; by the same token, they will reduce in size if you lose weight. Even non-reduced breasts have a tendency to droop a little through time and gravity, and you can expect a similar change in shape eventually to occur after a reduction operation. These provisos aside, you can continue to enjoy your new-found shape without fear.

I am a bra-size 38F, but a normal dress-size 10 everywhere else. I'm completely disproportionate and so I am having a breast reduction. I'd like a really petite bust, but is there any limitation to what they can do and how much they can take away?

This is an issue that you really must discuss with your surgeon before you undertake a breast-reduction procedure. A radical reduction is of course possible, but to achieve this goal, the shape and look of your breasts may be compromised. You may also end up with one breast a slightly different shape from the other.

In your case, where your bust is so disproportionately large in comparison to the rest of your petite frame, you may consider that the benefits of a significant reduction outweigh the possible imperfections of poor shape or a reduction in nipple function and sensitivity. But for women who have breasts that are only slightly larger than normal, these disadvantages need to be considered very carefully. ●

Breast reduction involves removing excess tissue, reshaping and repositioning the nipples. A radical reduction in size is possible but the shape may be compromised if too ambitious.

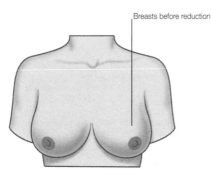

Breasts before reduction

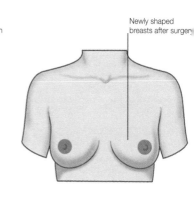

Newly shaped breasts after surgery

My daughter has told
me that she is going
to have a breast
reduction. I don't
want to stand in her
way, but I'm worried
for her. What are the
risks involved in such
a procedure?

There are undoubtedly some risks in a breast-reduction operation and these should be fully explained to your daughter before she agrees to the procedure. If they are not pointed out, then she should consider using a different surgeon.

As with any major operation involving an anaesthetic, there is a small risk of getting a chest infection, particularly among people who smoke. There is also a slight chance of getting a thrombosis in the veins of the leg, particularly among patients who are taking the contraceptive pill. In rare cases, heavy bleeding can occur after the operation and may mean a further operation or a blood transfusion.

Occasionally infection from germs harbouring in the ducts of the breasts may also cause problems. These can be successfully treated using antibiotics, but they do delay the healing process and sometimes result in scars needing to be restitched later. Usually the scars settle down well and end up as faint white lines, but in some cases the skin becomes flaky and forms a scab that separates to leave a broad scar. If you smoke, you increase the risk of this happening.

However, there is no evidence that reduction mammoplasty causes breast cancer; nor does it prevent you from examining your breasts for cancer in the normal way.

My best friend is saving up to have her breasts enlarged, but she seems to me to have very little information about the operation. She says she would rather not know, but I think it would be better if she were a bit more informed. What exactly should she expect from a breast-enlargement procedure?

Breast implants can be added through several different ways, in terms of both where the surgeon opens the breast and how the implant is placed, either above or under the chest muscle.

Breast-augmentation (or -enlargement) surgery consists of lifting the breast tissue and placing a natural-feeling implant either under the breast tissue or behind the chest muscle on which the breast lies. Usually an incision is made in the crease of the lower part of the breast, but sometimes incisions are made around the areola or in the armpit. Each of these methods is designed to leave minimal and discreet scarring. Once the incision is made, the implant is carefully placed in the breast and then adjusted for ideal size and symmetry, before the wound is sutured closed.

Your friend should be aware that she will need to wear a surgical dressing to protect the incisions and she will experience extensive swelling and bruising. The accompanying discomfort can be controlled with pain-relief medication. Her surgeon will let her know when she can get back to normal activity, but it will take some time for complete healing to occur. ●

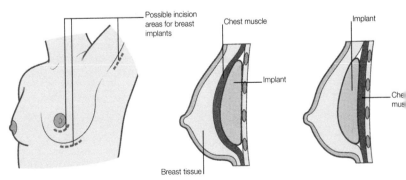

Possible incision areas for breast implants

Chest muscle

Implant

Implant

Che mus

Breast tissue

The complications and risks involved in a breast-augmentation operation are the same as those associated with all forms of surgery and anaesthesia. You should also add into the equation the possibility of additional problems, such as bleeding and infection.

In surveys as many as two-thirds of American women say that they are highly satisfied with their breast implants, but some women experience upsetting complications that may require further surgery or even removal of the implants. These include: implant rupture (where the implant contents leak into the surrounding tissue and even into other parts of the body); capsular contracture (whereby the fibrous tissue surrounding the implant distorts and shrinks, causing great pain); deflating saline-filled implants; and post-operative muscle spasms, causing pain.

Your surgeon will inform you of the probability of any of the above complications affecting you. For example, capsular contracture only occurs in about 10 per cent of patients and usually starts six or more months after surgery, and in some cases smoking increases the risk. Antibiotics and analgesic pain relief can readily treat problems such as infection and post-operative pain, but some problems may require the surgical removal of the implant.

I've heard bad things about silicone breast implants. My mother says she read that they can give you cancer. Is this true, and are any alternative implants available?

Your mother is quite right about the adverse media coverage given to silicone breast implants, but evidence now suggests that your fears are ungrounded. Undoubtedly there have been many changes and improvements to silicone implants since they were first introduced in 1963, and you will be relieved to know that breast-augmentation procedures have evolved considerably to lessen any post-operative complications.

Silicon is a naturally occurring element, which becomes silicone when it is combined with carbon, hydrogen and oxygen. Silicone is manufactured into many items, including cosmetics, foods and medical implants, and you will be hard pressed to avoid it, since just about all implants are made of an outer silicone shell, which the body tolerates quite well. The shell itself may be filled with silicone gel, salt water (saline solution) or soya-bean oil. The saline implant is now the one most commonly used.

Until the 1990s most implants contained silicone gel, which gave a more pleasing feel and natural look than today's saline implants. Over the years, however, this generated continued controversy, due to fears that silicone gel may have detrimental effects on the health of women with breast implants. There are currently more than 1.5 million American women with silicone breast implants, so as a matter of urgency numerous studies have now been carried out to establish the facts.

A comprehensive study by the American Institute of Medicine (IOM) focused on the major concerns in relation to the safety of silicone breast implants. They found evidence that clearly shows that silicone breast implants do not cause breast cancer or the recurrence of breast cancer. There is no evidence that silicone breast implants contribute to an increase in autoimmune (connective tissue) diseases. Examples of autoimmune diseases are *lupus erythematosus*, Raynaud's phenomenon, rheumatoid arthritis and scleroderma.

A report from the long-term Nurses' Health Study involving 87,505 women showed no link between implants and connective-tissue disease or rheumatic conditions. Annual studies agree, silicone-gel deposits are not a cause of neurological disease.

The IOM committee studied and evaluated multiple documents on the history, chemistry and toxicology of silicone implants. It noted that the wide use of manufactured silicone – in foods, cosmetics, lubricants and a variety of consumer products – had resulted in extensive exposure to it by individuals in all developed countries. The committee also concluded that the silicon found in tissues distant to the breast implants most likely reflects human exposure to the widespread presence of silicon and silicone in the environment and not just to the implants themselves.

At the end of its investigation the IOM committee concluded that the silicones found in breast implants do not represent a cause for concern at the doses that can reasonably be expected.

In addition the Independent Review Group, organized in the UK in response to women's concerns about silicone breast implants, concluded that, overall, the silicones found in breast implants were bland substances with little toxicity and no adverse effect on the body's immune system.

Q

63 I'm booked in for a breast-augmentation operation later this year, but I'm very anxious about the results. What if I don't like the shape of my new breasts once the operation is done?

The size and shape of your breasts after augmentation surgery is hard to predict and it will adjust with time. Taking that into consideration, it is probably best to keep a reasonably open mind about the final outcome. Breast implants can be round or anatomically shaped, and both give excellent results and have different merits that will be explained by your surgeon. Adjustable breast implants are also available that allow you to alter your breast size up or down within a certain time period following breast-augmentation surgery. This is particularly useful if you are dissatisfied with your shape after the operation. It also allows the surgeons to improve your breast shape and symmetry. The technique involves overfilling the implant to stretch the breast tissue, then removing some of the saline solution using a valve to obtain the final result.

Renewed clinical trials are also under way of a 'stacked' implant that has two compartments, each of which can be filled with a different volume. This allows the breast to achieve greater fullness at the base, with a gradual slope in the breast's upper portion. Initial trials in the mid-1980s looked promising, but were halted while the use of silicone implants was investigated. Although the US Food and Drug Administration (FDA) recently ruled that only one breast implant can be used in each breast, because the 'stacked' implant is a single device with two connected chambers it counts as one implant and thus does not contravene the FDA ruling.

Although the vast majority of women are pleased with the appearance of their breast implants, if you really did not like the effect, then as a last resort you could always have the breast implants removed. However, this is not to be recommended or undertaken lightly.

I'm not planning to
tell anyone, apart
from my nearest and
dearest, about my
planned breast
augmentation. But
how realistic will my
'new' breasts be, and
what can I expect
of them?

A good breast-augmentation operation should add pleasing dimensions to your overall proportion and symmetry. As long as you have not chosen an exceptional increase in breast size, there is no reason why people should suspect that your breasts are not natural. The latest implants achieve a very convincing look and feel, although there are some aesthetic and biological limitations.

Most women have slight asymmetry between their breasts and the operation can occasionally exaggerate this difference. And a breast that has an underlying implant will not necessarily feel exactly like a normal breast, although the silicone-gel implants have a more natural feel than the saline-filled ones. Another limitation is that it is not always possible to achieve a cleavage with breast augmentation, although this varies from patient to patient. Some women report that their breast implants look natural when they are standing, but that they don't look right when they are lying down.

Movement of the fluid that fills the implant may occasionally be seen through the skin – this is more likely to happen with the saline-filled implants rather than the more viscous silicone implants. However, this would not be noticeable through clothing, so you would only be at risk when sunbathing or wearing low-cut clothes. The early saline implants often created problems with 'deflation', but today's saline implants are much improved and deflation is now extremely rare.

The incisions for the operation are designed to leave minimal scarring. Nonetheless, breast augmentation will always leave some scars on the breast or in the armpit (*see Q 52*). The scars should not be detectable by the general public, but they will be obvious to you and your partner.

Having said all that, these are occasional or rare outcomes and most women with breast implants say that the overall effect and the psychological benefits of the procedure outweigh any such problems.

My sister's breasts felt unnaturally hard after she had her breast-enlargement operation and she experienced acute pain and discomfort. She eventually had her implants removed. Is this common?

Your sister is not alone in experiencing pain from her breast implants. Unfortunately the human body considers the implant to be a foreign agent and forms a protective capsule of fibrous tissue around it. This build-up of tissue is called a capsular contracture. In most cases the fibrous capsule around the implant does not pose any problems. However, if the build-up is severe, it can become painful and disfiguring as the capsule thickens and contracts, causing both the implant and the overlying tissue to distort. I don't know when your sister had her augmentation operation, but the newer implant designs have features inbuilt to reduce the likelihood of this occurring.

There are medical procedures to break down the overgrowth of protective tissue, including 'closed capsulotomy,' whereby strong pressure is applied to the outside of the breast to help break up the fibrous capsule. Sometimes the medical procedures are not sufficient and additional surgery to remove or replace the implants is required.

Problems with capsular contracture made up 28 per cent of secondary procedures done on women with breast augmentation and a recent study showed that it was the reason for 73 per cent of implant removals. However, placement of the implant behind the chest muscles seems to lower the chances of contracture occurring.

Q

66 I had a breast augmentation done about five years ago. At the time I was told that I would be able to breastfeed in the future. I am now married and we want to plan a family. Is it really safe – and indeed possible – to breastfeed with breast implants?

You can put your mind at rest: most women find that having a breast augmentation does not prevent them from breastfeeding, although some report that they have a slightly diminished milk supply. So give it a try – hopefully you will experience no problems.

There is absolutely no evidence of increased levels of silicon (see Q 62) being present in the breast milk of nursing mothers with implants. In fact, much higher levels of silicon (from which silicone is derived) have been found in cow's milk and commercially available infant formula than are found in the breast milk of women with implants.

In the past, concerns were also raised about the possibility of silicone crossing the placenta to the developing foetus in pregnant women with breast implants. However, the American IOM report found no evidence of increased levels of disease or birth defects in children born to women with implants.

I am 19 years old and I'm planning to have a breast-enlargement operation. Will this last me a lifetime?

Unfortunately it is unlikely that you will outlive your breast implants. The chances of having at least one replacement implant are high, and some women end up having many more.

In the US a study of women receiving reconstruction surgery over an average of six years showed that 16 per cent of those with saline implants required replacements. Another study reported an 18 per cent implant loss in women reconstructed with gel implants or submascular expanders (implants placed behind the chest muscle to help generate tissue growth in the breast area). As you get older, so the risks of having to undergo a replacement operation increase.

I have recently
found a breast
lump, which my
doctor says needs
further investigation.
However, he said that
my breast implants
might pose a
problem. What
did he mean?

Breast implants can interfere with a mammography, which is the X-ray screening method used to detect breast cancer (*see Q 86*). This is probably what prompted your doctor's remark. But special X-ray views can be taken to minimize this interference, and I am sure that your doctor will explain more fully if you ask him or her. Some types of implants do not interfere to such an extent, for example, soya-filled implants, so you should let your doctor and the mamogram technician know what type of implant you have.

There have also been reports that implants can interfere with radiation therapy. However, the findings of the American Institute of Medicine report suggest that implants show good stability in reaction to any necessary radiation doses, and that they do not interfere with radiation beams. Nonetheless, there is some mild cause for concern, in that radiation therapy may cause capsular contracture (shrinkage and distortion of the implant area (*see Q 65*)) and affect the feel and cosmetic look of your breasts. These issues should be discussed with your doctor or specialist before treatment.

Since I've had children my breasts have become very droopy. My husband says that I look fine, but I feel very self-conscious about them. Can anything be done to return them to their former glory?

There is a surgical procedure designed to combat the droopiness of breasts. When your breasts swell due to pregnancy and breastfeeding, the fibrous bands that support the breasts in their youthful shape start to break down and the skin stretches. As your breasts return to their normal size, the unsupported breasts settle into the stretched skin and gravity pulls them down.

Mastopexy (the uplifting of droopy breasts) reshapes the breast into a more youthful and firmer shape. During the procedure pleats of skin are removed from underneath the breast and the breast itself is remodelled into a tighter cone. The nipples are repositioned at a higher level so that they lie at the points of the tightened breasts; if desired, the size of the areola can be reduced as well. The best results are achieved with smaller sagging breasts, but any size of breast can be lifted, although results with a heavy bust may not last as long.

It is recommended that you seek mastopexy once your family is complete, so if you are planning to have any more children it may be wise to postpone the operation. That said, there is no risk to future pregnancy, and mastopexy does not necessarily interfere with breastfeeding. However, pregnancy is likely to stretch the breast again and reduce the efficacy of the procedure.

Sections of surplus skin are removed from underneath the breast.

Areolas can be reduced, making the nipples smaller and can make them seem more pert.

Nipples are repositioned further up the newly shaped breasts.

The scar line after a mammoplasty is usually round the areola of the breasts. This may cause a lack of sensation in the nipple area during sexual arousal.

Irrespective of your husband's kind comments, having perter, tighter breasts may well help your self-esteem. You should remember that although the appearance of your breasts will undoubtedly be improved, you will be left with scars and possibly some numbness in your nipples. Mastopexy can be carried out by a number of different techniques and the scars will differ accordingly. They are normally quite fine, but they are not invisible and could be noticeable if you were sunbathing topless, for example. ●

Q

70 **My friend went for a breast lift and came away with implants. How could this happen?**

Because the uplift procedure cannot re-create the natural attachment of the breast to the tissues underneath, mastopexy alone cannot increase the fullness of the breasts above the nipples. For this reason many women elect to have a breast implant to increase fullness while they are undergoing the mastopexy. However, this would not have been done without first discussing the issue with your friend or without her consent.

The only problem with having an implant to increase the size of the breasts is that the additional weight can accelerate the return of the droopiness that, unfortunately, is inevitable as time goes on. But your friend can lessen the rate at which this descent happens by supporting her breasts as much as possible in a well-fitted bra. ●

When things go wrong

Nine out of ten breast lumps are completely benign but the shock and fear of finding such a lump can be eased only through understanding the possible causes of such lumps, the procedures for diagnosing them and what happens if they are malignant. This section answers many of the most frequently asked questions about breast cancer.

Breast Cancer
& Treatment

Breast cancer is the most common cancer in women – the good news is that, should you be diagnosed with breast cancer, your outlook has never been better. At least half of all women in the UK who develop breast cancer are successfully treated and many others are able to live normal lives knowing that the disease is under control. This section explains the diagnostic procedures, and looks at the care and treatment now available for women.

71 What exactly is breast cancer, are we any nearer to discovering the causes of it and how can I tell if I have it?

Breast cancer is the second leading cause of cancer deaths in women (lung cancer being the first). It is also the primary cause of cancer deaths among women aged 35–54. Over the last 50 years the number of women diagnosed with the disease has increased each year.

Improvements in treatment and earlier detection with mammography have still only had a modest impact on the overall death rate, and new treatments have missed many of their targets. The majority of breast-cancer cases are 'sporadic' which means that there is no direct family history of the disease. Only 5–10 per cent of breast cancers occur in women with a clearly defined genetic predisposition to the

Breast cancer can take differing forms which vary in seriousness from hyperplasia in which cells within ducts multiply creating a benign tumour, to invasive carcinoma where malignant cells have spread to other areas of tissue.

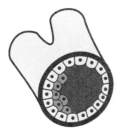

Hyperplasia

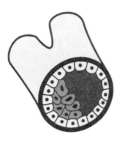

Atypical hyperplasia

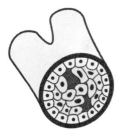

Cancer 'in situ'

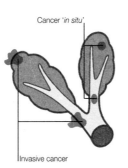

Cancer 'in situ'

Invasive cancer

disease. The overall risk of developing breast cancer increases as a woman gets older.

Cancer is caused by cells dividing inappropriately. Cells in the body usually only divide when new cells are needed, although occasionally they will divide for no reason, which creates a mass of tissue called a tumour. Cancer cells may also invade surrounding tissue or break off from a tumour and travel to other parts of the body, forming new tumours (a process known as metastasis); sometimes they travel through the lymphatic system or the blood vessels.

Nobody yet really understands why breast cancer occurs, although certain women do seem to have a greater risk of developing the disease. A small number of breast-cancer cases are genetic, and there are now special clinics for women concerned that they may have an increased risk of developing breast cancer. Women who have not had children or who had children late in life seem to have a marginally greater chance of getting breast cancer. Some evidence shows that women who eat a diet high in

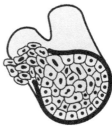

Invasive cancer

animal fat may also be at slightly higher risk. Taking hormone replacement therapy (HRT) for more than ten years may increase the risk, although this is still being looked into.

In the vast majority of women breast cancer is first noticed as a lump in the breast. Other signs may include changes in the size or shape of the breast, dimpling of the skin and lumpiness or thickening around the breast. Inverted nipples or a discharge or rash on the nipples may also be a symptom. Any swelling in the armpit should be checked out by your doctor in case the lymph nodes have been affected.

Breast cancer occurs in different forms and may be found early or after it has spread. Recovery depends on many factors, but early detection is the key to improving your chances of recovery. When found in its earliest stage, breast cancer is 90 per cent curable.

I have heard that only a tiny proportion of breast lumps turn out to be cancerous, but how can I tell which type I should worry about? I have found a fairly small lump in my breast. Should I bother my doctor or wait to see if it gets any bigger?

It is true that nine out of ten breast lumps are benign (not cancerous). However, if you do notice a lump in your breast you should get it checked out by your doctor, if only to set your mind at rest. It is always best to get any unusual symptoms examined, and your doctor will want to rule out the possibility of cancer. If it turns out that you do have cancer, then research shows that the earlier the treatment, the more successful it is.

If you are prone to lumpy breasts this does not mean you are more at risk of getting breast cancer. Six out of ten lumps in women under the age of 20 are known as fibroadenomas (see Q 14). Ultrasound and fine-needle aspiration are all that is usually required to confirm the diagnosis and you may find that you need no treatment at all. One in three of these types of lumps will get smaller or disappear of its own accord within two years.

Some women have breast cysts, which may start to form as you get older. They usually affect women between the ages of 30–50. Nobody knows what causes them, but most are smooth lumps that move around freely under the skin. Some are big enough to be clearly visible and may be painful. It is very easy to identify these cysts through ultrasound and mammography.

Benign lumps cause their own problems which can be treated and for your own peace of mind it is best to be sure.

LUMPS IN THE BREAST

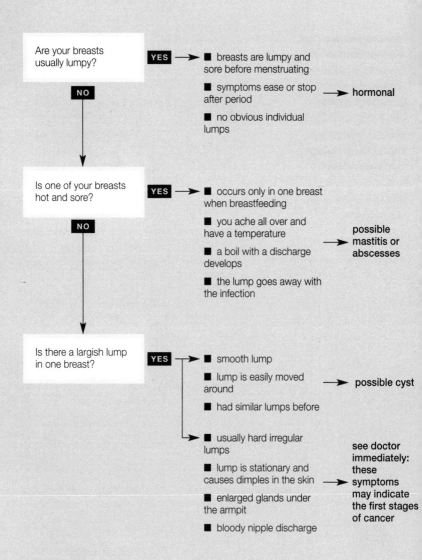

Are your breasts usually lumpy?

YES ➝ ■ breasts are lumpy and sore before menstruating

■ symptoms ease or stop after period ➝ **hormonal**

■ no obvious individual lumps

NO

Is one of your breasts hot and sore?

YES ➝ ■ occurs only in one breast when breastfeeding

■ you ache all over and have a temperature

■ a boil with a discharge develops ➝ **possible mastitis or abscesses**

■ the lump goes away with the infection

NO

Is there a largish lump in one breast?

YES ➝ ■ smooth lump

■ lump is easily moved around ➝ **possible cyst**

■ had similar lumps before

➝ ■ usually hard irregular lumps

■ lump is stationary and causes dimples in the skin ➝ **see doctor immediately: these symptoms may indicate the first stages of cancer**

■ enlarged glands under the armpit

■ bloody nipple discharge

Any lump in your breast should be checked by your doctor.

I have heard that having babies protects one against breast cancer and that there may be other ways in which one can reduce the risk of breast cancer. Is this true?

There are some factors that you can control to reduce your risk of breast cancer. Eating a balanced diet, restricting your alcohol intake to moderate levels, having an early first child and breastfeeding all add up to a good start.

Regular exercise also appears to reduce the risk of breast cancer. Researchers in California recently found that women who did four hours or more of exercise a week halved their risk of breast cancer. Just two hours of exercise a week – swimming, jogging, tennis or some other form of aerobic exercise – seemed to afford some protection. This seems to work by reducing levels of the female hormones that stimulate the breast cells.

There are women who are at very high risk of contracting breast cancer for whom other kinds of prevention may be advisable. Hormonal drugs used in the treatment of women who already have cancer may reduce by half the risk of contracting cancer. And occasionally women opt for a preventive mastectomy, when they are at extremely high risk. There is evidence that women who have their first baby when they are 30 have an increased risk of breast cancer. The reason is unknown, but one theory is that breast-cell changes that occur at the end of pregnancy might make cancer less likely.

I have been told that some hospitals operate a 'one-stop' breast-cancer clinic where you can have all the tests done and get the results the same day. Is this true and, if so, where can I get a list of such clinics?

It is true that some hospitals operate this type of clinic and the results are usually obtained the same day. You should be able to get a list of such clinics from your doctor or consultant (and *see page 138*). In a general hospital it will take longer for the results to come through and the waiting period can be an anxious time for you – it may help to talk through your worries with a partner, close friend or specialist counsellor.

Women report the best results for both breast-cancer diagnosis and treatment when they have been seen by a team of experts working together. Every woman is different and needs to think carefully about each type of treatment, working with doctors to develop the best approach for her.

I have heard that certain women are more at risk of getting breast cancer than others. Both my mother and my aunt had breast cancer. Does this mean that I will probably get it as well?

The good news is that 75 per cent of women with a family history of breast cancer will never develop the disease. Your increase in risk depends on how close the relative is and on how many relatives have had breast cancer. A woman whose mother developed cancer in both breasts before the age of 35, for example, has a 50 per cent chance of developing breast cancer herself. If both your mother and sister had breast cancer, you have

20 times the normal risk. If you have already had cancer in one breast, then you are at significantly higher risk, especially if your cancer occurred before the menopause.

It is generally believed that your risk of breast cancer increases as you grow older – about 70 per cent of women diagnosed with breast cancer each year are over the age of 50 and almost half are 65 or older. In women aged 40–49 there is a one in 66 risk and in the 50–59 age group the risk increases to one in 40. Your risk goes up if any relative developed breast cancer before the menopause, and if she had cancer in both breasts. Women with no family history of breast cancer are still at risk, particularly if they are over the age of 50. If you carry the familial breast-cancer gene (BRCA1 or BRCA2, see below) you are at very high risk.

Even distant family history, such as aunts, grandmothers and cousins, can increase your risk, although women with a family history of breast cancer account for only 5–10 per cent of all women with the disease.

Having your first child after the age of 30, or never having children, puts you at higher risk; the same is true if you started your period before the age of 12 or had a late menopause. Being overweight also increases your chances, as does a family history of any cancer, including cancer of the ovaries, cervix, uterus or colon. Two other factors include taking the contraceptive pill and HRT.

Q

76 What is the BRCA1
gene, and how do
I know whether or
not I have it?

BRCA1 was the first gene detected that was known to increase the risk of breast and ovarian cancer. The presence of this gene produces a greater than 90 per cent risk of developing such cancers by the age of 85. BRCA1 appears to account for about 45 per cent of familial breast cancers and 80 per cent of families with both breast and ovarian cancer. An estimated one in 600 women carries this gene. The risk of developing a second breast cancer among individuals carrying the BRCA1 gene is 65 per cent. Bilateral breast cancer is also common in women who carry this gene.

A second gene, BRCA2, also plays a major part in breast and ovarian cancer, although there is less information about the function of this gene. It is associated with an increased risk of ovarian cancer, and may account for a genetic link to male breast cancer. Both the BRCA1 and 2 genes can be inherited from either parent, so the father's family history of breast cancer is also important. Men or women who carry one of these gene mutations have a 50/50 chance of passing it on to their children.

In most people these genes help to prevent cancer by creating proteins that stop cells from growing abnormally. However, if a BRCA1 or 2 mutation (an alteration in genetic material) is inherited, then you may be more susceptible to developing cancer. In addition, women with an altered BRCA gene usually have an increased risk of developing breast cancer at a younger age (before the menopause). But not all women who carry these genes will develop cancer. At-risk families can take blood tests to screen for mutations in these genes, although genetic testing is done only when it is definitely indicated by a strong personal or family history. Genetic testing may also be used to determine whether a woman who has already been diagnosed with breast cancer is at an increased risk of getting a second breast cancer or ovarian cancer.

When someone with a cancer diagnosis and a family history of the disease has been tested and found to have an altered BRCA1 or 2 gene, the family is said to have a 'known mutation'. If an association between the development of breast cancer and a breast-cancer gene is made, then all family members willing to participate in genetic testing are asked to give a sample of blood. For many people, knowing their test results is important, because this information may help to guide health-care decisions for themselves and their families.

Does what I eat really make any difference, now that I know I have breast cancer?

Yes, it does. In fact, it is more important than ever to eat well when you have cancer. Eating nutritious food can help you feel better and have more energy, but you need to be aware that your calorie needs are different when you have cancer. Your estimated calorie needs are now about 15 calories per 1lb (0.454kg) of your own weight per day, if your weight has remained stable; add 500 calories per day if you have lost weight. For example, someone who weighs 150lb (68kg) needs about 2250 calories per day to maintain her weight. Eat plenty of protein that rebuilds and repairs body tissue. The best sources include dairy foods, meat, fish and poultry. You should also eat at least five portions of fresh fruit and vegetables per day.

Drink plenty of fluids: a minimum of eight glasses of fluid per day will prevent dehydration. That can include water, juice, milk, soup, milkshakes and other beverages. Tea and coffee don't count!

I have recently been diagnosed with breast cancer and can't help but worry about what is going to happen. Who will look after my children if I die, and what is the prognosis if I get better?

Your feelings are entirely normal for someone in this situation. There is nothing more stressful than being diagnosed with cancer and having to deal with the disease and all the 'unknowns' associated with it.

Women with breast cancer worry about how they are going to manage from day to day, as they struggle to keep up with the expectations of others. Rather than trying to maintain your normal daily routine, which may leave you exhausted, it may help to make lifestyle changes early on so that you can adapt and conserve your energy.

Help others to understand and support you – family and friends can only really be of assistance if they can 'put themselves in your shoes'. Cancer groups can be a good source of support as well, because other people who have had cancer will understand what you are going through. Relaxation techniques such as audio tapes that teach deep breathing or visualization can also help to reduce stress. And stress can easily turn into depression. One way to sort this out is to try to understand your depressed feelings and how they affect your life. If you are depressed all the time, were depressed before your cancer diagnosis or are preoccupied with feeling worthless and useless, then you may need treatment for depression.

79 Is there any
connection
between hormone
replacement therapy
and breast cancer,
and does taking the
pill increase the risk?

HRT has been shown to increase the risk of
developing breast cancer, especially after the
age of 60. Studies show that the risk is reduced when
HRT is stopped, and that it no longer increases about
five years after stopping. It also depends on how long
you take HRT – there is an increased risk if you take
it for more than ten years. The known link between
HRT and the risk of breast-cancer has discouraged
many women from choosing this treatment, and
most specialists do not recommend HRT for breast-
cancer survivors.

However, women at risk of cardiovascular disease
are four times more likely to die from heart problems
as from breast cancer, and HRT has been shown to
reduce the risk of developing heart disease by up to
50 per cent. It also substantially reduces the risk of
osteoporosis (which causes weakness of the bones).
Some doctors therefore believe that the benefits of
oestrogen-only HRT in preventing cardiovascular
disease and osteoporosis are worth the risk, even in
high-risk women.

The latest HRT treatments are known as selective
estrogen receptor modulators (SERMs) and appear to
protect against the development of breast cancer, as
well as increasing bone density. Recent studies show
that some SERMs reduce the risk of breast cancer in
post-menopausal women by 70 per cent.

As far as the pill is concerned, 150 million women have used the contraceptive pill since its introduction 40 years ago. None of the research studies to date has produced any evidence that there is a substantially increased risk of breast cancer in women who take the pill, although of course some women with breast cancer have been on the pill and among women who have a family history of breast cancer the pill may cause a slight increase in risk. The only types of contraceptive pill that have been controversial are ones that contain oestrogen, as this hormone is known to have a link with breast cancer. The progesterone-only pill carries no risk at all.

I feel very ambivalent about my breast cancer and am not sure that I really want to have all the treatment. What would happen if I took a risk and just carried on living a normal life? Might the cancer cure itself?

It would be wrong of you to forego all treatment for your breast cancer. However, that does not mean that you don't have a right to deal with your cancer in any way you see fit. And if that means you don't want to go through invasive treatment, then that must be your decision. There have been cases of women who have had breast cancer and have made miraculous recoveries, but these cases have been very few and far between. It is a risk you take. There are some holistic treatment centres where they believe that each individual has her own resources and insight that she brings to bear on the recovery process. They aim to help you harness those, and your inner strength, through an holistic approach.

81 I have a lump in my breast, which has worried me for a few weeks now. How can my doctor tell if I have breast cancer, and what procedures can I expect to go through?

There are certain warning signs that your doctor will look for, which may signal breast cancer. These include a lump (which might be as small as a pea) or any sort of thickening of the breast tissue or in the underarm area that persists throughout the menstrual cycle. Your doctor will also be watching out for any change in the size, shape or contour of the breast or any blood-stained or clear fluid discharge from the nipple. Any change in the feel or appearance of the skin on the breast or nipple, such as dimpling or puckering, might also ring warning bells. Such changes are often found by the woman herself while performing monthly breast self-examination. That is why it is so important to check your breasts every month, so that you become familiar with the normal monthly changes in them.

When you first report a lump to your doctor he or she will examine you to see whether you need to have any tests and x-rays. If you are referred to a specialist you will be asked for your medical history, and your breasts will be examined for any sign of enlarged lymph glands under your arms and at the base of your neck. A chest x-ray and blood tests may also be taken to find out the state of your general health. Other tests may include a mammography (see Q 86)or ultrasound scanning. Ultrasound is normally recommended to find out whether a lump is solid or contains fluid. A special gel is spread onto the breasts and a small hand-held device that emits soundwaves is passed over the area. The echoes are then converted by a computer into pictures of the inside of the breast tissue. The whole procedure is painless and takes just a few minutes.

I have been told that I have ductal carcinoma. I know it's cancer, but what does it mean?

There are several different types of breast cancer, named because of where they start initially and the pattern they follow as they spread in the breast.

The two most common types of breast cancer are ductal carcinoma (which starts in the lining of the milk ducts of the breast) and lobular carcinoma (which begins in the lobules of the breast, where breast milk is produced).

In the first instance ductal carcinoma refers to cancer that is confined to the milk ducts and has not invaded nearby breast tissue. If left untreated, ductal carcinomas *in situ* may become invasive cancer in the long-term and spread throughout the breast. Whilst serious in itself lobular carcinoma *in situ* also serves as a marker showing the increased risk of developing breast cancer in both breasts.

Cancers can form in other parts of the breast, but these are more rare. If you are at all unsure about anything to do with your cancer you should ask your doctor for as much information as you want.

My doctor has told me that I am to be sent for a needle aspiration. Is this an operation, and what does it involve?

This is not an operation, but a quick and simple procedure that is usually done in the outpatients' clinic. It is normally recommended when a woman has presented with a breast lump. Using a fine needle and syringe, a doctor takes a sample of cells from the breast lump and sends it off to the laboratory to see whether it contains any malignant cells. This technique may also be used to drain a benign cyst. Sometimes, particularly when the lump is small, a needle aspiration may be carried out in the x-ray department. The doctor then uses a x-ray or ultrasound guidance to ensure that a specific area of the breast is sampled with a special needle before sending the sample off to be tested.

The fine needle aspiration examination can be carried out in an outpatient clinic. It involves the insertion of a fine needle into the breast lump to remove a few of the suspect cells for laboratory testing.

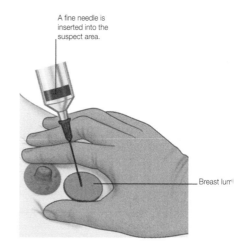

A fine needle is inserted into the suspect area.

Breast lump

My friend recently had breast cancer and she was shocked at the incredible number of different tests that had to be done before she knew what was wrong and what treatment she would need. What are these tests, and why do they have to be done?

Your friend is not alone in being bewildered by the number of tests you have to undergo to diagnose and treat breast cancer.

First, you will see your own doctor, who makes the initial diagnosis after a thorough examination of your breasts. During the breast exam, the doctor carefully feels the lump and the tissue around it. Cancerous lumps usually feel different in size and texture from benign lumps. When abnormal tissue is found during an examination or a mammogram, a small sample of cells or tissue is removed from the affected area using surgery, needles or other techniques – this is known as a biopsy.

After the sample is removed, it is sent to a laboratory for testing. A pathologist views the sample under a microscope and looks for abnormal cell shapes or growth patterns which show if the cells are cancerous. If cancer is present, the pathologist can tell what kind of cancer it is and whether it is invasive and has spread beyond the ducts or lobules. Laboratory tests, such as hormone-receptor tests, can also show whether the cancer is sensitive to hormones which helps your doctor to decide on types of treatment. Positive test results mean that certain hormones help the cancer to grow, so the cancer is likely to respond to hormone treatment to counteract this effect.

If the tests show that you have breast cancer, the doctor may want to do further tests to establish whether there has been any spread of the disease. These can help the doctor decide on the best type of treatment for your particular cancer. The tests may include blood tests, X-rays and sometimes bone and liver scans. It is only through as much knowledge as possible that the doctor can work out the best treatment plan for your cancer. ●

85 Throughout my life I have had lumpy breasts and they have never given me cause for concern. However, now that I am in my late forties I have been told I need a triple-assessment test. What does this actually mean, and what does it involve?

Being advised by your doctor to have a triple-assessment is not something you should worry about, and is probably based on your age rather than a natural tendency to lumpy breasts. Studies show that the earlier breast cancer is diagnosed the more successfully it is treated, so by being cautious your doctor is safe-guarding your health.

The triple-assessment itself involves a clinical examination, some kind of imaging of the breast (such as mammography or ultrasound) and taking some tissue for examination under the microscope. If the results of all three tests are negative you will be sent home with the all-clear. Otherwise, further tests may be needed, which may include surgical removal of the lump.

Whatever the case, you will be given the chance to discuss all the treatment options before undergoing surgery or any other treatment. ●

My friend told me that when she had a mammogram recently it was really painful. Is it true that your breasts are squeezed between two flat pieces of metal, and can't the radiation harm your breasts?

There is no point beating about the bush. A mammogram is not particularly pleasant. Although the procedure is described as 'painless', most women say it is at best uncomfortable and at worst agony! But the sensation lasts no more than 10 or 15 seconds, so it is usually bearable.

A mammogram is a low-dose X-ray of the breast that can pick up small cancers and other abnormalities, which neither you nor your doctor can feel on manual examination. You will be asked to strip to the waist and stand in front of the machine while the radiologist compresses your breast between two plates. The radiographer takes two views of each breast and you are normally given the results a few days later. Some women are concerned about these low levels of X-rays, but the tiny risk of them actually causing you any harm is far outweighed by the benefits of detecting breast cancer early on. ●

A mammogram works by compressing each breast under a perspex paddle in order to see through the breast tissue. Any abnormal lumps can then be seen on the resulting x-ray picture.

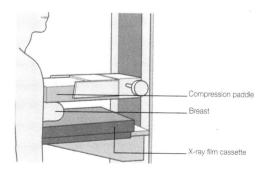

Compression paddle

Breast

X-ray film cassette

87 I have recently been diagnosed with breast cancer and I find all the jargon associated with the disease really confusing. What is invasive ductal carcinoma, for example, and how does it differ from invasive lobular carcinoma and hyperplasia?

During your fertile life the glands and ducts in the breasts are in a permanent state of growth, development and shrinkage.

Ductal carcinomas (*see Q 82*) account for more than 80 per cent of all detected breast cancers. The first symptom is normally a new hard, ill-defined lump within the breast. As the tumour spreads along the strands of connective tissue between the breast lobes, it pulls on the overlying skin, causing a dimpling effect. This extreme skin pitting is a serious sign, which means that the cancer has become invasive. Invasive lobular cancer accounts for about 10 per cent of breast cancers and may spread rather diffusely, rather than forming a tumour. 'Hyperplasia' describes the overgrowth of cells in any part of the lobes or ducts. While hyperplasia always implies a benign condition it does carry a small increase in the risk of contracting cancer. Actual cancer comes at the far end of the hyperplasia spectrum. This 'spectrum' covers the overgrowth of cells which usually goes through four distinct phases. Firstly, they start to multiply more than necessary, secondly, they lose their normal appearance, thirdly, these atypical cells fill up the duct forming a carcinoma and fourthly, they become invasive carcinoma. This is when these atypical cells break out of the duct and spread to the surrounding tissues.

I have heard that mammograms are not all they are cracked up to be, but my doctor has told me that, now that I am over 50, I should have one. Is the procedure really necessary, or are there any other screening techniques that I could ask for?

Mammograms are not 100 per cent foolproof, as a small number of breast cancers do not show up on them. It is also less effective in women under the age of 50, since their breast tissue is more dense and abnormalities do not show up as well. However, this is still a more sensitive procedure than a simple manual breast examination. Studies in Sweden and the USA have shown that screening can reduce deaths from breast cancer in women between the ages of 50 and 65 by up to one-third. Early detection means early treatment which increases the chances of full recovery if breast cancer is found. As such, it is an excellent diagnostic tool to investigate and look for breast lumps.

Ultrasound is good for examining dense breasts, especially where breast cysts may be suspected. It is therefore good for younger women and can detect much smaller lumps which cannot yet be felt. It produces a picture made from the echoes of soundwaves bouncing off tissue.

Thermography produces heat sensitive photographs and is rarely a first line investigation but usually requires a mammogram and manual examination as backup. It works by mapping out tissue temperatures using infra-red photography so a growing cyst or tumour will show up as a more intense area of heat than the surrounding tissue.

89 Recently I was diagnosed with breast cancer. Is all treatment the same and, if so, what treatment am I likely to have?

Once you are diagnosed with breast cancer you and your doctor will develop a treatment plan within a few weeks. That plan will be as much about treating the cancer as about reducing the chances of it returning. Your doctor will use a variety of tests to discover how aggressive the tumour is, the stage of the disease and whether it has spread. Once these factors have been determined, you and your doctor will be able to decide on the best form of treatment for your cancer and can assess your long-term outlook. The type of treatment you receive will depend on the size and location of the tumour in the breast, the results of laboratory tests done on the cancer cells and the extent of the spread of the disease.

Breast-cancer treatments range from surgery and radiation to systemic treatments (which are used

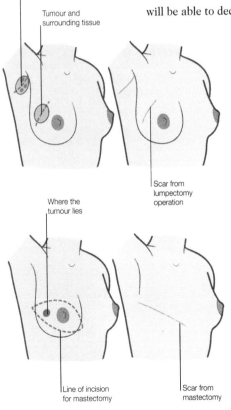

Lymph nodes

Tumour and surrounding tissue

Scar from lumpectomy operation

Where the tumour lies

Line of incision for mastectomy

Scar from mastectomy

The type of operation performed will depend on the size, extent and location of the tumour in the breast.

to destroy or control the cells), including chemotherapy (see Q 99) and hormone therapy. You may have just one form of treatment or a combination, depending on your wishes and needs.

Breast surgery ranges from a lumpectomy to a total mastectomy. Lumpectomy involves cutting away the cancerous portion of the breast, and an area of normal tissue surrounding the cancer, while striving to preserve the normal appearance of the breast. Some of the lymph nodes under the arm may also be removed. Treatment is usually followed by six to eight weeks of radiotherapy (see Q 99) to treat the remaining breast tissue. Most women who have a small, early-stage tumour respond well to this type of surgery and post-operative treatment.

Mastectomy, or removal of part of or the entire breast, is another option (see Q 92). The mastectomy procedures performed today are not the same as the older, radical mastectomies, which involved removing the breast tissue, skin and chest-wall muscles. Modern procedures do not usually remove the muscles and, for many women, they are accompanied by either immediate or delayed breast reconstruction. What happens after surgery depends on whether your doctor thinks there is a likelihood that the cancer will recur. Certain types of breast cancer require oestrogen to grow so hormone treatments such as Tamoxifen work by blocking the action of oestrogen in a woman's body. This is not foolproof and is used alongside other treatments.

90 My friend has just been diagnosed with breast cancer, but has been told it is at stage 1, so does this mean she can relax? What exactly are the different stages, and what do they mean?

There are several stages of breast cancer with each stage being more invasive and complicated to treat.

Stage 1 breast cancer is normally defined when a tumour smaller than, or equal to, 2cm (¾in) in diameter is diagnosed, but the underarm lymph nodes test negative for cancer. Stage 2 is either when a tumour larger than 2cm (¾in) is diagnosed and the underarm lymph nodes test negative for cancer, or a tumour smaller than 5cm (2in) is diagnosed but the underarm lymph nodes test positive for cancer.

Stage 3A breast cancer is defined as a tumour larger than 5cm (2in) with lymph nodes that test positive for cancer, or any-sized tumour with cancerous lymph nodes that stick to one another or to surrounding tissue. Stage 3B indicates a tumour of any size that has spread to the skin, chest wall or internal mammary lymph nodes (found below the breast and inside the chest). Stage 4 is a tumour of any size that has spread to places far away from the breast, such as the bones, lungs or lymph nodes.

Advanced breast cancer which is comprised of stages 3 and 4 is defined as when the cancer cells have spread to the lymph nodes and to other parts of the body. Recurrent breast cancer is when the disease has returned despite initial treatment. Recurrent cancer too can then go through the above stages.

Both stages 1 and 2 may be curable by surgery alone, although they may require chemotherapy or radiotherapy as well. At stage 3 the cancer has invaded the muscles of the chest wall, the overlying skin and possibly even the lymph nodes, and by stage 4 the cancer has spread to several other parts of the body; the outlook at this stage is poor. As a rule of thumb, the five-year survival rate of 85 per cent of stage-1 tumours falls to less than 10 per cent for stage 4. It is through diagnosis and consultation with your doctor that a cancer comes to be fully understood in its growth pattern and a treatment plan is worked out.

Each stage of breast cancer becomes more invasive and difficult to treat which is why so much emphasis is on finding the tumours at the earliest stage possible through self-examination and mammograms.

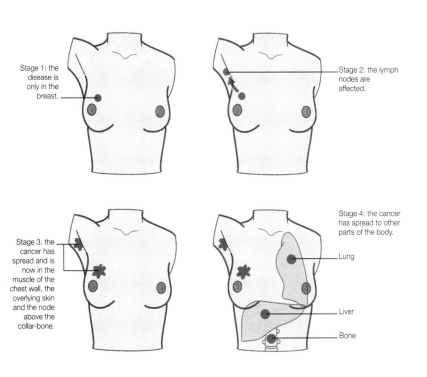

Stage 1: the disease is only in the breast.

Stage 2: the lymph nodes are affected.

Stage 3: the cancer has spread and is now in the muscle of the chest wall, the overlying skin and the node above the collar-bone.

Stage 4: the cancer has spread to other parts of the body.

Lung

Liver

Bone

91 I recently discovered a lump in my breast that I now know is malignant, and I am terrified of losing both my breasts. What is the current thinking about treatment: do they try to save the breast at all costs? I have also heard about partial mastectomy, but what does this involve?

The current approach to breast cancer is to conserve as much of the breast as is feasible by performing the least possible amount of surgery. If your lump is less than 4cm (1½in) in diameter, for example, you should be suitable for a lumpectomy, which is emotionally far less traumatic than a mastectomy and is better cosmetically. This operation is carried out under general anaesthetic and you may have to stay in hospital for four to five days to make sure that the scar heals and there are no complications.

A partial mastectomy involves removing part of the breast: the cancer, along with some of the surrounding tissue. Segmental excision (or quadrantectomy) is a similar procedure, but involves removing more tissue in the area of the breast that is involved. This means that it may be more noticeable, particularly in women who have small breasts. Depending on how much tissue is removed, these operations can leave a misshapen breast, and some women prefer to opt for a total mastectomy.

A radical mastectomy is very rare these days, but removes the muscles on the chest wall as well. A modified radical mastectomy removes the breast and lymph glands, leaving the chest-wall muscles intact. In any breast-cancer operation the surgeon usually removes lymph glands from under the arm so that he can check whether any cancer cells have spread from the breast and establish whether any other treatment is needed. Some surgeons remove all the armpit lymph glands, while others take just a few lymph glands as a representative sample.

I am booked in to have a mastectomy and am keen to get up and about as soon as possible after my operation. What can I realistically expect, and will I experience a lot of pain?

Whatever type of operation you have had you will be encouraged to get out of bed and start moving around as soon as possible after the operation. You may have a drainage tube running from the wound, but this is usually removed by the nurses a few days after the operation. Some women are allowed home with the drainage tube still in place, in which case it will be removed a few days later by a community or district nurse.

After the operation you will have some pain or discomfort, which may continue for some weeks. Painkilling drugs can be very effective. If you have had a mastectomy you will be given a lightweight foam prosthesis, which you can start wearing inside your bra. It is specially designed to be worn straight after the operation, when the area is still feeling tender. When you return home it is best to take things easy for a while. You may feel physically and emotionally exhausted, so try to get plenty of rest and eat a well-balanced diet. You may be advised not to lift or carry anything heavy and you should not drive a car for at least four weeks.

The doctors have caught my cancer early on, so I am going to have a lumpectomy. I have heard that with this procedure, and with mastectomy, you lose all sensation in the nipple. Is this true?

A lumpectomy is the usual option for many women at your stage and involves the removal of the breast lump together with some of the surrounding tissue. It removes the least possible amount of breast tissue, but leaves a small scar and sometimes a tiny dent in the breast. For most women, the appearance of the breast after a lumpectomy is very good, and they may require a hospital stay of only a few days. It is not usual to lose sensation in the nipple after this operation.

What you have heard about is the numbness, tingling or stiffness that you often feel in your upper arm as a result of this operation. This occurs if the surgeon has removed lymph nodes from under your arm, or if you have had radiotherapy to the armpit and the nerves in the area have been affected by the treatment. These side-effects may last for some months but are rarely long-term. However, it is extremely rare for a lumpectomy to cause loss of sensation in the nipple.

Your consultant will refer you to see a physiotherapist, who will teach you some simple exercises to ensure that you recover movement and normal feeling as soon as possible. It is important to do these exercises regularly so that you regain the movement in your arm. ●

I am so grateful that doctors have found my breast cancer early, although I am still going to lose one of my breasts. I don't know yet how I am going to feel after the op, but would like to know more about breast reconstruction so that I can make up my mind about it at a later date. Am I likely to be turned down if I want this operation?

It is now quite common for women to have a breast reconstruction done at the same time as a mastectomy. The outcome for her, both physically and psychologically, has been proven to be better. If you are keen to have breast reconstruction you should discuss it with your doctor at the beginning of your treatment, so that he or she can tell you about the different methods available. If your doctor is reluctant to consider this option, you should seek a second opinion.

Your breast (including your nipple) will be refashioned, using either an implant or your own fat and muscle by means of a 'flap' operation. Expander implants are usually a first step towards a permanent implant. Increasing amounts of fluid are injected into the expander bag over a period of time until enough space has been created for the permanent implant to be inserted.

BREAST RECONSTRUCTION

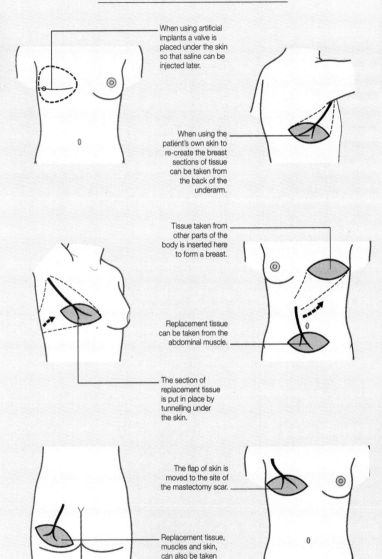

When using artificial implants a valve is placed under the skin so that saline can be injected later.

When using the patient's own skin to re-create the breast sections of tissue can be taken from the back of the underarm.

Tissue taken from other parts of the body is inserted here to form a breast.

Replacement tissue can be taken from the abdominal muscle.

The section of replacement tissue is put in place by tunnelling under the skin.

The flap of skin is moved to the site of the mastectomy scar.

Replacement tissue, muscles and skin, can also be taken from the buttocks.

I found a lump in my breast three years ago and the surgeons successfully removed it. I feel 100 per cent healthy and have got back on with my life, but there is a niggling part of me that worries that it could return. What is the likelihood, and when can I feel I am really 'cured'?

If you have survived breast cancer, this is such a natural concern. There are many organizations to help women who have or have had breast cancer, your doctor will be able to give you some addresses (see page 138).

You must remember that the longer you live free of a recurrence, the better are your chances of a complete cure. Most doctors believe that you should be carefully monitored for at least five years to detect possible recurrences or secondary spread of the disease. However, if you are symptom free for ten years or beyond without a recurrence or spread, then you can consider yourself cured.

I have been having regular radiotherapy following surgery for breast cancer and now my skin has started to itch and burn. What does this mean, and is it normal?

Please don't worry – this is a completely normal reaction to radiotherapy. During your treatment radiation passes through your skin, so it is hardly surprising that you have had some reactions to it. Your skin may become red, swollen, warm and sensitive (just as if you have sunburn); it may peel, or become moist and tender. Such skin reactions are common and temporary: they generally subside gradually within four to six weeks of completing treatment. If skin changes appear outside the treated area, inform your doctor immediately.

Long-term side-effects, which can last up to a year or more after treatment, may include a slight darkening of the skin, enlarged pores on the breast, increased or decreased sensitivity of the skin, a thickening of breast tissue or skin, and a change in the size of the breast.

You can reduce skin reactions by gently cleansing the treated area using luke-warm water and a mild soap. Do not rub your skin, but pat it dry with a soft towel or use a hair-drier on a cool setting.

Do not scratch or rub the treated area and do not apply any ointment, cream, lotion or powder to it unless your radiation oncologist or nurse has either prescribed it or signalled their approval.

Try and avoid tight-fitting clothing or clothes made from harsh fabrics, such as wool or corduroy, which are more likely to irritate your skin. Instead, choose clothes made from natural fibres such as cotton and linen.

Do not expose the treated area to extreme heat or cold, and avoid getting it in direct sunlight, which may make your skin reaction worse and lead to a bad case of sunburn. Choose a sunblock/sunscreen of SPF 15 or higher, and protect yourself from direct sunlight even after your course of treatment has been completed.

You can ask your doctor for more specific advice about skin treatments and sun protectors.

It is now more than three months after my surgery and chemotherapy for breast cancer. I knew I might feel tired after the operation, but I can hardly keep my eyes open in the afternoons. Is this normal, and is there anything I can take to help?

Cancer-related fatigue (CRF) is one of the most common side-effects of cancer and its treatment. Usually it comes on suddenly, and many women describe it as 'paralysing'. The exact reason for CRF is unknown, but any chemotherapy drug can cause fatigue. Some women find that the fatigue lasts a few days, while others say the problem persists throughout the course of treatment and even after it is over. Radiotherapy can also cause cumulative fatigue, which usually lasts for three to four weeks after treatment stops, but may continue for up to two or three months.

Any tumour can cause what is known as 'hypermetabolic' state. This is because cancerous cells compete for nutrients, often at the expense of normal cells' growth. In addition to fatigue, weight loss and decreased appetite are common side-effects.

Cancer treatments can also cause reduced blood counts leading to anaemia, which is in turn known to cause fatigue. Anaemia is a blood disorder in which there is too little haemoglobin in the blood. Haemoglobin is a substance in the red blood cells that enables the blood to transport oxygen throughout the body and, when the blood cannot transport sufficient oxygen, the result is extreme and sometimes debilitating fatigue.

Q

98 **Since losing one of my breasts to breast cancer two years ago, I can't bear my husband to touch me. We have tried talking and he is incredibly understanding, but I don't feel I am a woman any more. Would counselling help?**

Yes. Many women who have lived through the experience of breast cancer have found counselling extremely helpful. The diagnosis of breast cancer is a very traumatic experience for most women. No two individuals are the same, but many women describe feeling shocked, anxious and angry. Some women also say that they lose their self-confidence, particularly with regard to feelings of loss of attractiveness and femininity. It is understandable that you may feel ambivalent about your body as a result of losing your breast. Loss of confidence and a change in the way you see yourself can also affect your sexual relationship.

Many hospitals have a breast-care nurse who can provide support and information. She can also talk to your husband and family, if they are finding it difficult to adjust. Some women prefer to talk to other women who have had breast cancer. Most countries have a nationwide network of women who offer this service, and there are also self-help and support groups (*see page 138*). ●

What exactly is the difference between chemotherapy and radiotherapy? Why do they make you feel sick, and do they always cause your hair to fall out?

Chemotherapy involves using a combination of drugs that kill off, or slow down, the growth of rapidly multiplying cancer cells. There are many drug combinations used to treat breast cancer and they are given either intravenously or orally. Once they enter the bloodstream, they travel to all parts of the body so that they do not miss any cancer cells that may have spread beyond the breast itself.

Chemotherapy is given in cycles of treatment followed by a recovery period. The entire treatment generally lasts three to six months, depending on the type of drugs given. Chemotherapy is often given after a lumpectomy or mastectomy and is then known as adjuvant treatment. This type of treatment can help to reduce the risk of the disease recurring. Chemotherapy is sometimes given before surgery in order to shrink a tumour so that it can be more easily removed or so that a lumpectomy (rather than a mastectomy) can be performed. It may also be given as the main treatment for women whose cancer has spread to other parts of the body beyond the breast and lymph nodes.

The side-effects of chemotherapy depend on the type and amount of medication you are given and how long the treatment lasts. Not everybody experiences side-effects, so if you do not have any this does not mean that your treatment is not working. The most common side-effects include nausea and vomiting, loss of appetite, hair loss, mouth sores, changes in the menstrual cycle or a premature menopause. You are also at higher risk of infection (due to decreased white blood cells), bruising or bleeding and fatigue. Most people can continue to work while they are being treated with chemotherapy, and you may be able to schedule your treatments for later in the day or at the weekend so that they don't interfere with your work too much.

Radiotherapy uses high levels of radiation to kill cancer cells or keep them from growing and dividing. Radiation is delivered to the affected breast and, in some cases, to the lymph nodes under the arm or at the collar-bone.

Radiotherapy is usually given after a lumpectomy (and sometimes after a mastectomy) to reduce the chances of the disease coming back. The treatments generally start several weeks after surgery so that the area has some time to heal. Once radiotherapy treatment starts, you can expect to receive small daily doses of radiation over a period of several days to several weeks. When you go for treatment the radiotherapist will take you into a treatment room, where you will be helped onto a table and asked to lie in the correct treatment position. Once she is sure you are positioned correctly, she will leave the room and start the radiation treatment, during which time you will be under constant observation. It is important to remain still and relaxed during treatment; the machine will not touch you and you will feel nothing during the process. Once your treatment is complete, the radiographer will help you off the treatment table.

During treatment radiation passes through your skin, so one of the side-effects is a change in the skin area exposed to radiation, which may become dry, red and itchy. Radiotherapy does cause nausea in some cases, but will not cause your hair to fall out. 🌸

My mother had a radical mastectomy, which left her pretty much unable to move or lift anything. She used to love exercising and longs to go back to the gym. Are there any gentle exercises she could do?

Even during cancer therapy it is often possible to continue exercising. If you keep up your physical activity levels you will conserve your energy and not feel so tired. Regular, moderate exercise will also stop you from feeling depressed.

Your mother should check with her doctor before beginning any exercise programme, but the main thing for her to remember is to start slowly and allow her body time to adjust. Most exercises are safe, as long as she proceeds with caution and does not overdo it.

The safest and most productive activities to start with are swimming, and walking, she can then progress slowly on to more energetic exercises such as indoor stationary cycling and low-impact aerobics. Providing she is careful these activities carry little risk of injury and benefit her entire body. 🌸

Useful Information

FURTHER READING

Pregnancy and breastfeeding

THOMAS, PAT, *The Common Sense Approach to Pregnancy*, Newleaf, 2001

Breastfeeding: Avoiding Some of the Problems, National Childbirth Trust, 1992

GOTSCH, GWEN, *Breastfeeding Pure & Simple*, La Leche League International, 1999

NAISH, FRANCESCA, and ROBERT, JANETTE, *The Natural Way to a Better Pregnancy*, Newleaf, 2000

NAISH, FRANCESCA, and ROBERT, JANETTE, *Healthy Lifestyle, Better Pregnancy*, Doubleday, Australia, 1999

HOGG, KAREN, et al., *Breastfeeding Your Baby*, Thorsons, 1998

KITZINGER, SHEILA, *Breastfeeding*, Dorling Kindersley, 1998

LOTHROP, HANNAH, *Breastfeeding Naturally*, Fisher Books, 2000

MORAN, ELAINE, *Bon Appetit, Baby! The Breastfeeding Kit*, Treasure Chest Books, 2000

PALMER, GABRIELLE, *Politics of Breastfeeding*, Pandora, 1988

RENFREW, MARY, et al., *Bestfeeding: Getting Breastfeeding Right for You*, Celestial Arts, 2000

ROYAL COLLEGE OF MIDWIVES, *Successful Breastfeeding*, Churchill Livingstone, 1999

SEARS, WILLIAM, MD, *The Breastfeeding Book: Everything You Need to Know About Nursing Your Child from Birth Through Weaning*, Little, Brown, 2000

SMALE, MARY, *The National Childbirth Trust Book of Breastfeeding*, Vermilion, 1999

ENGEL, JUNE, *The Complete Breast Book*, Newleaf/Key Porter, Toronto, 2000

TUCKER, FELICITY, 'Practical Parenting' Problem Solvers: Breastfeeding, Pan, 1999

Breast cancer

FALLOWFIELD, LESLEY, and CLARKE, ANDREW, *Breast Cancer*, Routledge, 1991

GRIGG, MARTHA, *Breast Cancer and You: Bettering the Odds*, Branden Books, 1995

HIRSCHAUT, YASHAR, and PRESSMAN, PETER I., *Breast Cancer: The Complete Guide*, Bantam Books, 2000

LANGE, VLADIMIR, *Be A Survivor: Your Guide to Breast Cancer Treatment*, Lange Productions, 1999

LATOUR, KATHY, *The Breast Cancer Companion*, Avon Books, 1994

LINK, JOHN, MD, *The Breast Cancer Survival Manual*, St Martin's Press, 2000

OLIVIER, SUZANNAH, *The Breast Cancer Prevention and Recovery Diet*, Penguin, 2000

SAMPSON, VAL, and FENLON, DEBBIE, *The Breast Cancer Book*, Vermilion, 2000

UDALL, KATE GILBERT, *Breast Care: The Woman's Guide to Cancer Prevention and Optimal Breast Health Through Nutrition and Lifestyle*, Woodland Publishing, 1999

WADLER, JOYCE, *My Breast: One Woman's Cancer Story*, Women's Press, 1994

WITTMAN, JULIET, *Breast Cancer Journal: A Century of Petals*, Fulcrum Publishing, 1993

Breast surgery

DIXON, MICHAEL, et al., *Operative Breast Surgery*, Churchill Livingstone, 2000

ENGLER, ALAN M., MD, *BodySculpture: Plastic Surgery of the Body for Men and Women*, Hudson Publishing, 2000

HEASMAN, MAXINE KAYE, *The Ultimate Cleavage: A Practical Guide to Cosmetic Breast Enlargement Surgery*, M. Heasman, 1999

STEWART, MARY WHITE, *Silicone Spills*, Praeger Publishers, 1998

STUMM, DIANA, *Recovering from Breast Surgery: Exercises to Strengthen Your Body and Relieve Pain*, Hunter House Inc., 1995

VANDERFORD, MARSHA L., and SMITH, DAVID H., *The Silicone Breast Implant Story*, Lawrence Erlbaum Associates, 1996

Pregnancy and breastfeeding

Association of Breastfeeding Mothers
26 Holmshaw Close
London SE26 4TH
tel: 020 8778 4769

La Lèche League (Great Britain)
BM 3424
London WC1N 3XX
tel: 020 7242 1278
La Lèche League of Ireland
tel: 1 282 9638

National Childbirth Trust
Alexandra House, Oldham Terrace
London W3 6NH
tel: 020 8992 8637

Homebirth Association of Ireland
36 Springlawn Court
Blanchardstown, Dublin 15

Women's Health Queensland Wide
PO Box 665
Spring Hill 4004, Australia
tel: 3839 9988(in Bris)
1800 017 676 (rest Qld)

Family Planning ACT
Health Promotion Centre
Childers Street, GPO Box 1317
Canberra ACT 2601, Australia
tel: (02) 6247 3077
education phone: (02) 6247 3018
e-mail: fact@familyplanningact.org.au

Irish Family Planning Association
Unity Building
16/17 Lr O'Connell Street, Dublin 1
tel: 1 878 0366
website:
http://www.ifpa.ie

Breast cancer

Breakthrough Breast Cancer
A research charity committed to
discover the causes, preventions and
treatments for breast cancer.
tel: 0207 405 5111
website:
http://www.breakthrough.org.uk

**Breast Cancer Care (formerly the
Breast Care and Mastectomy
Association for Great Britain)**
helplines: 0500 245 345 (London) and
0141 221 2233 (Glasgow)

British Association of Cancer United Patients (BACUP)
Gives advice and information on all aspects of cancer, as well as emotional support for individuals affected by breast cancer and their families and friends.
information: 0207 696 9003 (London) and 0800 181199 (outside London)

Cancer Care Society (CARE)
Offers counselling, emotional support and practical information, rather than medical support, for patients, their families and friends.
tel: 0117 942 7419

Macmillan Cancer Relief
15–19 Britten Street
London SW3 3TZ
Has a list of specialist breast units and specialist breast surgeons in the UK; write to them for a copy.

Women's Nationwide Cancer Control Campaign (WNCCC)
Campaigns for early detection and prevention; produces a nationwide clinic list for anyone wanting to find her nearest clinic.
tel: 0207 729 2229.

Breast Cancer Action Group NSW
BGAG NSW Inc.
PO Box 5016,
Greenwich NSW 2065, Australia
website: www.users.bigpond.com

The Cancer Association of South Africa
website:
http://www.cansa.org.za
email: cansainfo@cansa.org.za

The Irish Cancer Society
5 Northumberland Road
Dublin 4
Ireland
tel: 1 668 1855
website:
http://www.irishcancer.ie

Reach to Recovery (Ireland)
A support group for breast cancer sufferers contactable through The Irish Cancer Society
tel: 1800 200 700

Breast Cancer Online

An independent educational service and information source for professionals working in the field of breast cancer. It includes conference information and reports, news, links, case studies and questions for self-assessment.

website: http://www.bco.org

Community Breast Health Projects

Offers information to patients and survivors of breast cancer. It includes practical advice and links to other websites that have breast-cancer information.

website: http://www-med.stanford.edu/CBHP/

National Alliance of Breast Cancer Organizations (NABCO)

A coalition of more than 370 organizations that provide breast-cancer detection, treatment and care to thousands of women. The site gives information on clinical trials, a resource route to cancer-information services on the Internet and links to local breast-cancer support groups.

website: http://www.nabco.org/

Y-ME National Breast Cancer Organization

Has a commitment to provide information and support to anyone who has been affected by breast cancer. The site includes general information about breast cancer, screening and detection; information for both women and men who have breast cancer; and information for family members and loved ones.

website: http://www.y-me.org/

OTHER USEFUL SITES

http://www.breastcancerfund.org
http://www.irishcancer.ie
http://www.cansa.org.za
http://www.breast-cancer-research.com
http://www.canceranswers.org
http://www.cancerguide.org
http://www.cancerhelp.com
http://www.cancernet.nci.nih.gov
http://www.Cancernews.com

British Association of Aesthetic Plastic Surgeons (BAAPS)
The Royal College of Surgeons of England
35–43 Lincoln's Inn Fields
London WC2A 3PN
tel: 020 7405 2234
website: http://www.baaps.org.uk
e-mail: info@baaps.org.uk

British Association of Plastic Surgeons (BAPS)
The Royal College of Surgeons of England
35–43 Lincoln's Inn Fields
London WC2A 3PN
tel: 020 7831 5161
website: http://www.baps.co.uk
e-mail: secretariat@bas.co.uk

Colleges of Medicine of South Africa
17 Milner Road
Rondebosch 7700
tel: 27 21 689 3161
website:
http://www.collegemedsa.ac.za

Association of Plastic and Reconstructive Surgeons of Southern Africa
website:
http:www.plasticsurgeons.co.za

Australian Society of Plastic Surgeons
Level1, 33-35 Atchinson Street
St Leonards 2065
Sydney
Australia
tel: 1 300 367466
website:
http://www.asps.asn.au

Royal College of Surgeons in Ireland
123 St Stephen's Green
Dublin 2
tel: 1 402 2100
website:
http://www.rosi.ie

Further information on the safety of silicone breast implants can be found at the following website:
http://www.nap.edu/catalog/9618.html

Index

ACKNOWLEDGEMENTS

The authors would like to thank the following organizations for their help in compiling the information for this book: www.cosmeticsurgery.org and www.baaps.org.uk websites